ANNALS *of* THE NEW YORK ACADEMY OF SCIENCES

T0179752

EDITOR-IN-CHIEF
Douglas Braaten

ASSOCIATE EDITOR
Rebecca E. Cooney

PROJECT MANAGER
Steven E. Bohall

EDITORIAL ADMINISTRATOR
Daniel J. Becker

Artwork and design by Ash Ayman Shairzay

The New York Academy of Sciences
7 World Trade Center
250 Greenwich Street, 40th Floor
New York, NY 10007-2157

annals@nyas.org
www.nyas.org/annals

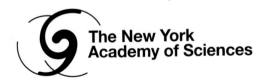

**The New York
Academy of Sciences**

Published by Blackwell Publishing
On behalf of the New York Academy of Sciences

Boston, Massachusetts
2011

ANNALS *of* THE NEW YORK ACADEMY OF SCIENCES

VOLUME
1245

ISSUE

Animal Models: Their Value in Predicting Drug Efficacy and Toxicity

This volume stems from the conference "Animal Models and Their Value in Predicting Drug Efficacy and Toxicity," which was jointly presented by the Global Medical Excellence Cluster and the New York Academy of Sciences, in collaboration with the Centre for Integrative Mammalian Physiology and Pharmacology at Imperial College London and King's College London. The conference was generously supported by Bronze Sponsors, GlaxoSmithKline, Pfizer, sanofi-aventis, the Global Medical Excellence Cluster, and the Wellcome Trust; and also by Academy Friend Sponsors, Bristol-Myers Squibb, the British Pharmacological Society, Charles River, Imperial College London, King's College London, the National Swine Research and Resource Center, Sigma Advanced Genetic Engineering (SAGE Labs), Taconic, the Jackson Laboratory, and the Physiological Society. Additional funding was made possible, in part, by the Office of the Director of the National Institute of Environmental Health Sciences (NIEHS), Grant R13RR032638 from the National Center for Research Resources (NCRR), the National Institute of General Medical Sciences (NIGMS), and the National Institute of Diabetes and Digestive and Kidney Diseases (NIDDK).

The views expressed in written conference materials or publications, and by speakers and moderators, do not necessarily reflect the official policies of the U.S. Department of Health and Human Services, nor do mention by trade names, commercial practices, or organizations imply endorsement by the U.S. Government.

TABLE OF CONTENTS

1   Have animal models of disease helped or hindered the drug discovery process?
Ann Jacqueline Hunter

3   Current models and strategies in the development of antiobesity drugs
James S. Kinsey-Jones and Kevin G. Murphy

7   Relevance of angiotensin II-induced aortic pathologies in mice to human aortic aneurysms
Dennis Bruemmer, Alan Daugherty, Hong Lu, and Debra L. Rateri

11   Novel, nonreflex tests detect analgesic action in rodents at clinically relevant concentrations
Nick Andrews, Sinead Harper, Yasmin Issop, and Andrew S.C. Rice

14   Animal welfare and the 3Rs in European biomedical research
Dominic J. Wells

17   Best practices for the use of animals in toxicological research and testing
William S. Stokes

Become a Member Today of the New York Academy of Sciences

The New York Academy of Sciences is dedicated to identifying the next frontiers in science and catalyzing key breakthroughs. As has been the case for 200 years, many of the leading scientific minds of our time rely on the Academy for key meetings and publications that serve as the crucial forum for a global community dedicated to scientific innovation.

 Select one FREE *Annals* volume and up to five volumes for only $40 each.

 Network and exchange ideas with the leaders of academia and industry.

 Broaden your knowledge across many disciplines.

 Gain access to exclusive online content.

Join Online at **www.nyas.org**

Or by phone at **800.344.6902** (516.576.2270 if outside the U.S.).

21 Progress toward generating informative porcine biomedical models using induced pluripotent stem cells
Franklin West and Steven Stice

24 A knockout mouse resource for the biomedical research community
K.C. Kent Lloyd

27 Minimizing strain influences in a genetically modified mouse phenotyping platform
Michael D. Hayward, Olesia Buiakova, and David S. Grass

31 The blessings and curses of C57BL/6 substrains in mouse genetic studies
Camron D. Bryant

34 Modeling inflammation and microvascular dysfunction
Felicity N.E. Gavins

36 TRPV1 and TRPA1 channels in inflammatory pain: elucidating mechanisms
Susan D. Brain

38 Imaging of endocrine gene expression in a humanized transgenic rat
Julian R.E. Davis

40 Systems biology of the heart: hype or hope?
T. Alexander Quinn and Peter Kohl

44 Is it time for *in silico* simulation of drug cardiac side effects?
Gary R. Mirams and Denis Noble

48 Human stem cell-derived cardiomyocytes for pharmacological and toxicological modeling
Sian E. Harding

50 Humanized mice as a preclinical tool for infectious disease and biomedical research
Leonard D. Shultz, Michael A. Brehm, Sina Bavari, and Dale L. Greiner

55 Humanized mice for the study of type 1 and type 2 diabetes
Dale L. Greiner, Michael A. Brehm, Vishnu Hosur, David M. Harlan, Alvin C. Powers, and Leonard D. Shultz

59 Deconstructing hepatitis C virus infection in humanized mice
Marcus Dorner and Alexander Ploss

63 Animal models got you puzzled?: think pig
Eric M. Walters, Yuksel Agca, Venkataseshu Ganjam, and Tim Evans

Online only

Systems Pharmacology of Complex Diseases
Jens Hansen, Shan Zhao, and Ravi Iyengar

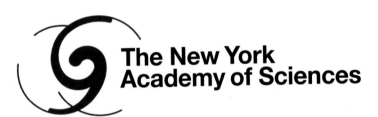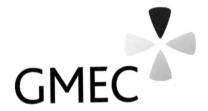

In Collaboration with The Centre for Integrative Mammalian Physiology and Pharmacology at Imperial College London, and King's College London

Ann. N.Y. Acad. Sci. ISSN 0077-8923

ANNALS OF THE NEW YORK ACADEMY OF SCIENCES

Issue: *Animal Models: Their Value in Predicting Drug Efficacy and Toxicity*

Have animal models of disease helped or hindered the drug discovery process?

Ann Jacqueline Hunter

OI Pharma Partners Ltd. Weston, Herts, United Kingdom

Address for correspondence: Ann Jacqueline Hunter, Ph.D. OI Pharma Partners Ltd, Red Sky House, Fairclough Hall, Halls Green, Weston, Herts SG4 7DP, UK

Animal models have played an important role in target validation, screening of compounds for efficacy and optimization of pharmacokinetic properties and toxicological testing. However, new paradigms for drug discovery and development will require a greater emphasis on animal models of mechanism.

Keywords: drug discovery; preclinical models

Over the past decade there has been a realization that the current model for drug discovery and development is becoming more unsustainable. This is reflected in the fact that the costs of drug discovery and development have doubled over the past decade, yet new medicine approvals have remained static. The major reasons for compound failure are lack of efficacy in patients and unexpected toxicity.[1,2] The failure of positive data in animal models of disease to translate into meaningful data in the clinic has led researchers and others to question the validity of these models. This has been especially true for areas such as the central nervous system (CNS), where animal models are perceived to be less predictive of the human condition, although recent data on failures in phase II trials across therapeutic areas does not necessarily show that the CNS is worse than some other therapeutic areas.[3]

In the past, many of the animal models that predicted the efficacy of compounds in the clinic were symptomatic in nature, for example, models where the effects on blood pressure were measured, and chemically induced seizures in normal mice were used to study the effects of anti-convulsants. Disease models did exist, such as those for cancer, stroke and pain, and these were used for screening, although they were not necessarily more predictive than the symptomatic models. With the advent of the completed human genome sequence, there was an enormous rise in the number of genetic models

of disease, primarily in mice, as well as a focus on developing new models of disease based on human physiology. However, these advances in model development have not made a significant increase in improving the rate of success in phase II proof-of-concept studies. So what can we do to better utilize animal models to develop new medicines, especially for the treatment of complex diseases?

There are actually very few models of human disease in animals that faithfully reproduce all aspects of the human pathophysiology and symptomatology. This is not surprising, as most human diseases are highly heterogenous. There are many good models of particular aspects of a disease, for example, an individual pathological feature or symptom. This does not devalue a model, providing the limitations in terms of extrapolating any findings to the whole patient population are recognized and acknowledged. An example is the G39A SOD transgenic mouse model of ALS, which uses a mutation that is responsible for only a very small percentage of ALS patients.[4] Although the model is relatively rapid and mimics the symptomatology and some aspects of the pathology, key pathological changes are missing. Even with this very specific model, there are important differences between laboratories in terms of measurements, reproducibility and drug effects. Significant variability between experiments within a lab can also occur, and positive effects in this model have failed to translate into clinical

doi: 10.1111/j.1749-6632.2011.06375.x

benefit.[5] Perhaps of greater concern is that molecules that failed to work in this ALS model have not progressed to the clinic, and this is also true in other areas where there is great variability in the disease models, for example, multiple sclerosis (MS).

For all disease models, whether surgically or pharmacologically induced or genetic, there needs to be clarity around the pathology that is being modeled in the animal and how it relates to the human condition. For example, in stroke research the ability of a drug to produce neuroprotection relies on the stroke model having sufficient collateral blood flow in the compromised infarcted area for the compound to be able to reach the cells and halt cell death. Likewise, such neuroprotective compounds should only be taken into clinical populations where there is a perfusion/diffusion mismatch, that is, in patients who have a compromised area that is still salvageable.[6]

It is also important that the right molecules are taken into the clinic—some failures that have been attributed to a failure of a particular animal model may actually have been due to the fact that the compound tested clinically had not been demonstrated for target exposure, target engagement, and/or pharmacological activity at the target. Where there is often little or no agreement across researchers about which is the most appropriate animal model for a disease, it can be hard to estimate the required exposure at the target for activity based on the disease models. This is because the concentrations (exposures) of a compound in preclinical models required for efficacy can differ across the various models used, even when these models are carried out in the same laboratory. This complexity makes it difficult to extrapolate the exposures necessary for efficacy in human patients.[7]

With the advent of more target validation in humans through genetic and other studies, it is timely to embrace new models of drug development: ones where animal models still play a key role, but where there is more focus on animal models of *mechanism*, rather than animal models of *disease*. What do I mean by a model of mechanism? For example, if a compound is thought to have potential in MS, say via blocking the influx of leukocytes into the brain and hence suppressing neuroinflammation, then demonstrating that the compound causes this blockade in animals might alone be sufficient for progression to humans. Demonstrating that such blockade of influx happens in phase I studies in the clinic should give confidence to move the molecule into phase II studies. Hence, would there be any need to show an effect in the mouse experimental autoimmune encephalomyelitis (EAE) model of MS? Such a mechanistic approach is frequently used with antibodies where there is no activity at the rodent target, as there are few primate models of disease. Ideally, the focus should be on developing mechanistic *in vivo* assays that can be translated to humans—assays that can demonstrate that a compound affects the target mechanism, give an understanding of the exposures required for efficacy on the mechanism, allow comparison of pharmacodynamics with pharmacokinetics, and hopefully advance molecules to the clinic more rapidly.

Conflicts of interest

A.J.H. is an ex-employee and shareholder of GlaxoSmithKline PLC; a nonexecutive director and shareholder with Proximagen Group PLC; and CEO and owner of OI Pharma Partners Ltd.

References

1. Pammolli, F., L. Magazzini & M. Riccaboni. 2011. The productivity crisis in pharmaceutical R&D. *Nat Rev Drug Discov.* **10:** 428–438.
2. Paul, S.M., D.S. Mytelka, C.T. Dunwiddie, *et al.* 2010. How to improve R&D productivity: the pharmaceutical industry's grand challenge. *Nat Rev Drug Discov.* **9:** 203–214.
3. Kola, I & J. Landis. 2004. Can the pharmaceutical industry reduce attrition rates? *Nature Drug Discov.* **3:** 711–714.
4. Montes, J., C. Bendotti, M. Tortarolo, *et al.* 2008. *Translational research in ALS in Animal and Translational models for CNS drug discovery, Vol 2.* R.A. McArthur & F. Borsini, eds.: 267–297. Academic Press.
5. Schanbel, J. 2008. Standard Model. *Nature* **454:** 682–685.
6. Albers, G.B. 1999. Expanding the Window for Thrombolytic Therapy in Acute Stroke: The Potential Role of Acute MRI for Patient Selection. *Stroke* **30:** 2230–2237.
7. Valenzanoa, K.J., L.G. Tafesseb, G. Leeb, *et al.* 2005. Pharmacological and pharmacokinetic characterization of the cannabinoid receptor 2 agonist, GW405833, utilizing rodent models of acute and chronic pain, anxiety, ataxia and catalepsy. *Neuropharmacology* **48:** 658–672.

Ann. N.Y. Acad. Sci. ISSN 0077-8923

ANNALS OF THE NEW YORK ACADEMY OF SCIENCES

Issue: *Animal Models: Their Value in Predicting Drug Efficacy and Toxicity*

Current models and strategies in the development of antiobesity drugs

James S. Kinsey-Jones and Kevin G. Murphy

Section of Investigative Medicine, Department of Diabetes, Endocrinology and Metabolism, Hammersmith Campus, Imperial College London, London, United Kingdom

Address for correspondence: Kevin G. Murphy, Section of Investigative Medicine, Department of Diabetes, Endocrinology and Metabolism, Hammersmith Campus, Imperial College London, Du Cane Road, United Kingdom. k.g.murphy@imperial.ac.uk

Animal models have enabled investigation of the complex mechanisms underlying energy homeostasis and, therefore, the development of antiobesity drugs.

Keywords: obesity; animal model; antiobesity

Obesity is one of the greatest challenges currently facing healthcare systems across the world, with more than 1.5 billion people overweight and over 500 million of these being clinically obese.[1] Obesity has been linked with increased risk of several chronic diseases including type 2 diabetes, cardiovascular disease, and certain cancers.[2] Furthermore, the economic cost of obesity-associated diseases is estimated to be $100 billion per year in the United States alone.

The increasing prevalence of obesity is believed to be driven primarily by the increased availability of high-fat (HF) energy-dense food and a progressively more sedentary lifestyle. Obesity is the result of a sustained imbalance between energy intake and expenditure, where a surplus of energy results in increased body weight. One therapeutic solution is a combination of diet and exercise. However, although this remains the most successful nonsurgical treatment of obesity, poor adherence and regain of lost weight remain significant problems.[3] Bariatric surgical procedures are the most effective treatments for obesity, resulting in sustained weight loss and improvement or resolution of comorbidities. However, financial cost, perioperative risk, and limited availability of surgical expertise and resources prevent it from acting as a panacea for the obesity epidemic. For example, although laparoscopic banding has recently been approved for individuals with a BMI >30 kg/m^2 with comorbidities, it seems unlikely that there are the available resources to carry out this surgery on the 27 million Americans who are eligible for it.[4]

Another treatment option for obesity is pharmacotherapy. At present, there is a profound disconnect between the prevalence of obesity and the availability of drug therapies. There are only two U.S. Food and Drug Administration (FDA)–approved drugs available for the treatment of obesity: phentermine and orlistat. Phentermine, an appetite suppressant, was approved by the FDA in 1959, but only for short-term use because of concerns regarding long-term safety. Orlistat inhibits the absorption of dietary fat, and, thus, results in a moderate reduction in body weight and, frequently, unpleasant gastrointestinal side effects. Unfortunately, antiobesity drugs have an unfortunate history of poor safety profiles and low efficacy. The reasons for these difficulties likely lie in the complex systems, which regulate energy homeostasis. Although there are many potential therapeutic targets involved in these systems, there are also potentially many counter-regulatory systems that may be activated by pharmacological interventions. In addition, many target molecules regulate other physiological systems besides energy homeostasis. There is clearly a pressing need to develop effective and safe new therapies. Animal models are an important component of the research programs needed to develop such agents.

doi: 10.1111/j.1749-6632.2011.06343.x

Table 1. Comparison of rodent obesity models

Animal model	Example	Strengths	Limitations
Diet-induced obesity (DIO)	High-fat diet	Similar physiology to human obesity. Responsive to clinically effective drugs.	Variation induced by different rodent strains and diets. Expensive to generate.
Monogenetic obesity	*ob/ob*, lacking leptin	Well characterized, produces robust obese phenotype.	Deficient in leptin signaling: a pivotal regulator of energy homeostasis. Does not reflect the majority of human obesity.
Polygenic obesity	New Zealand obese (NZO) mouse	Use in examining the contribution of genetic factors in obesity: natural genetic variation. Majority of human obesity polygenic.	Difficult to identify the genetic basis for the phenotype. Major differences between different polygenic models.
Knock-out (KO) models	Melanocortin 4 receptor-KO	Can provide insight into specific energy homeostasis–regulating genes.	Developmental compensations and nonspecific effects.

Animal models of obesity have provided the cornerstone of our understanding of the physiological and genetic basis of obesity. Although nonhuman primates, dogs, and seasonal mammals have been used, rodents are the most extensively studied animal models in obesity research. There are a number of reasons why these phylogenetically distant animals provide good models for human obesity. Like humans, rodents are omnivores and have complex taste and digestive systems for identifying and consuming a variety of different foods. Second, the neuroanatomy of rodent feeding circuits is similar to that of humans. In addition, antiobesity agents have largely been found to produce similar effects on food intake and body weight in laboratory rodents and humans.[6]

A number of different types of animal models are used in obesity-drug discovery (Table 1). Selecting the correct model is critical and often dependent on the mechanisms through which candidate drugs mediate their actions. To study acute effects on food intake is often easier using a paradigm by which basal food intake is elevated. This is most commonly achieved by an overnight fast. This methodology has the advantage of being simple. It can be used to rapidly obtain data regarding the efficacy, potency, duration of action, and any potential side effects of a novel agent. However, fasting is a stressor that activates the hypothalamic-pituitary-adrenal axis (HPA),[5] which may modulate the actions of certain drugs on food intake. Further, examining acute food intake is not a useful way to assess the efficacy of drugs that may reduce body weight by increased energy expenditure or reduced nutrient absorption. Chronic models of food intake allow the long-term effects of such agents to be studied, and are also used to determine whether a drug target can alter food intake in freely feeding animals, and thus under more physiological conditions. Chronic models also provide important information about whether the anorectic effects observed in acute studies can be sustained, and whether they can drive a reduction in body weight.

Chronic studies are often conducted in obese animals, which can be generated through either dietary or genetic manipulations. Diet-induced obesity (DIO) models are the result of providing a normal rodent with a HF diet for three to four months. These animals exhibit an increased body weight, largely caused by increased body fat. The changes observed in DIO rodents mimic many of those observed in obese patients: insulin resistance, elevated plasma leptin, cholesterol, and triglyceride levels. Importantly, such DIO models are sensitive to clinically effective weight loss agents. For example, administration of the cannabinoid-1 receptor antagonist Rimonabant reduces body weight in DIO mice and rats, and this effect is mirrored in humans.[6] Together, these data suggest the presence of common biological pathways in both DIO rodent models and human obesity. However, there can be large differences in the responses to HF diet between mouse strains. Indeed, certain strains of mice and rats demonstrate a resistance to body weight gain when exposed to a HF diet, such models are known as dietary-resistant strains. Careful consideration is, therefore, needed when selecting the strain to use. In addition, DIO animal models are generated through a regimen whereby the animals are exclusively fed on a HF diet. When given the choice, different mice strains display different preferences in dietary fat content (ranging between 28% and 83% of total energy).[7] Most humans have a choice of foods, though many enjoy and, therefore, choose to preferentially eat HF diets. An individual's susceptibility to obesity may, thus, be derived from an innate preference for HF foods. Such complex human food selection behaviors can be difficult to reflect in animal models. However, animal models have been used to elucidate the complex neuronal circuitry underlying the food reward system, including such potential antiobesity targets as the dopamine mesocortico–limbic system.

Genetic models of obesity have provided great insights into the mechanisms underlying the control of food intake and the dysregulation of these systems that can occur in obesity. Spontaneous monogenic mutations have given rise to some of the best characterized models of obesity, for example, the leptin signaling–deficient mice (*ob/ob*, *db/db*) and Zucker rats (*fa/fa*). These obese animals display hyperphagia, hyperinsulinaemia, and hyperlipidaemia. However, the absence of an intact leptin system creates such a powerful drive to eat in these animals that it may mask potentially effective anorectic agents. Indeed, antiobesity agents that are effective clinically or in DIO animals have attenuated effects in animals lacking leptin or its receptor.[6] Single-gene mutations only account for a small minority of human obesity. Polygenic models of obesity have, therefore, been suggested to more accurately replicate the human disease. Such models

can be generated from selective breeding programs in which animals exhibiting a number of traits such as rapid weight gain are selected. However, other traits that are inadvertently also selected during this process may make comparison between strains difficult.

Transgenic mice have greatly increased our understanding of the pathways regulating appetite, and, thus, of potential therapeutic targets. For a number of obesity targets, knock-out (KO) phenotypes and the effects of drugs acting at the same target are complementary. KO models can be used to assess the potential off-target actions of specific drugs. However, although genetically modified mice are useful to identify potential therapeutic targets and to demonstrate the mechanisms by which such agents work, the interpretation of their phenotypes requires careful evaluation. Many KO models have altered energy homeostasic phenotypes, but this can reflect nonspecific effects or developmental roles rather than a physiological role in the regulation of energy homeostasis in adult animals.[8] In addition, developmental compensation can occlude the actual role of potential obesity targets. To circumvent or reduce the effects of potential compensatory mechanisms, conditional KO systems incorporating spatial and/or temporal control of gene functions can be used.

Though there is much academic and industrial research interest in obesity, there is a dearth of new obesity drugs entering the clinic. One reason for this failure is the importance of safety to the success of agents in the drug development pipeline. Any pharmaco-therapy for obesity will likely have to be administered chronically, possibly for the remaining life of the patients. Using a combination of agents at lower individual doses may result in fewer side effects. A combination of obesity drugs may, therefore, prove a more effective treatment than targeting a single system. For example, administration of topiramate or phentermine alone only modestly reduces body weight in DIO rats. Coadministration, however, induces a more robust decrease in body weight, and similar effects are observed in humans.[6] Over recent years, agents based on gut hormones have shown promise as novel antiobesity therapies. Gut hormones play a vital physiological role in the regulation of appetite and body weight. Gut hormones are released peripherally and act relatively specifically on the central circuits that regulate food intake, which may mean that they have fewer or less severe side effects than drugs that target central neurotransmitters or ubiquitous receptor systems. Indeed, administration of specific gut hormones to animal models and to man has been shown to result in short-term weight loss. Interestingly, bariatric surgery, the only effective therapy for long-term weight loss, has been shown to increase circulating levels of anorectic gut hormones. It is possible that the effects of such surgery on body weight are, at least, partly mediated by changes in a number of gut hormones, which may act additively to reduce appetite and body weight. Combinatorial strategies are now being used in the development of gut hormone therapies.[9] Administering a combination of drugs on the basis of a number of different anorectic gut hormones may mimic natural satiety mechanisms and the changes observed after bariatric surgery, and therefore provide an effective antiobesity treatment.

In summary, animal models have provided great insight into the etiology of human obesity. Hopefully, the targets identified and investigated using such models will lead to the development of much needed antiobesity drugs in the future.

Conflicts of interest

The authors declare no conflicts of interest.

References

1. World Health Organization. 2011. Obesity and overweight fact sheet No 311.
2. Kopelman, P.G. 2000. Obesity as a medical problem. *Nature* **404:** 635–643.
3. Wadden, T.A., M.L. Butryn & C. Wilson. 2007. Lifestyle modification for the management of obesity. *Gastroenterology* **132:** 2226–2238.
4. Eckel, R.H., S.E. Kahn, E. Ferrannini, *et al.* 2011. Obesity and type 2 diabetes: what can be unified and what needs to be individualized. *J. Clin. Endocrinol. Metab.* **96:** 1654–1663.
5. Adam, T.C. & E.S. Epel. 2007. Stress, eating and the reward system. *Physiol. Behav.* **91:** 449–458.
6. Vickers, S.P., H.C. Jackson & S.C. Cheetham. 2011. The utility of animal models to evaluate novel anti-obesity agents. *Br. J. Pharmacol.* **164:** 1248–1262.
7. Smith, B.K., P.K. Andrews & D.B. West. 2000. Macronutrient diet selection in thirteen mouse strains. *Am. J. Physiol. Regul. Integr. Comp. Physiol.* **278:** R797–805.
8. Reed, D.R., M.P. Lawler & M.G. Tordoff. 2008. Reduced body weight is a common effect of gene knockout in mice. *BMC Genet.* **9:** 4.
9. Field, B.C., A.M. Wren, V. Peters, *et al.* 2010. PYY3–36 and oxyntomodulin can be additive in their effect on food intake in overweight and obese humans. *Diabetes* **59:** 1635–1639.

Ann. N.Y. Acad. Sci. ISSN 0077-8923

ANNALS OF THE NEW YORK ACADEMY OF SCIENCES
Issue: *Animal Models: Their Value in Predicting Drug Efficacy and Toxicity*

Relevance of angiotensin II-induced aortic pathologies in mice to human aortic aneurysms

Dennis Bruemmer, Alan Daugherty, Hong Lu, and Debra L. Rateri

Saha Cardiovascular Research Center, University of Kentucky, Lexington, Kentucky

Address for correspondence: Alan Daugherty, Saha Cardiovascular Research Center, Biomedical Biological Sciences Research Building, B243 University of Kentucky, Lexington, KY 40536-0509. Alan.Daugherty@uky.edu

Angiotensin II infusion in mice promotes abdominal and thoracic aortic aneurysms, which provides a feasible approach to study the mechanisms of these two distinct diseases.

Keywords: aortic aneurysms; angiotensin II; mouse; human

Introduction

Abdominal aortic aneurysms (AAAs) and thoracic aortic aneurysms (TAAs) are two distinct human vascular diseases that are not only distinguished by different locations but also by different etiologies. For example, AAAs have strong positive associations with aging, male gender, and smoking but have relatively weak genetic associations.[1] In contrast, many forms of TAAs may occur in early life with no sexual dimorphism and have strong genetic components, as exemplified by Marfan's syndrome and other hereditary diseases.[2] As there are no validated medical therapies for either AAAs or TAAs, treatment is restricted to open or endovascular surgical repair. Therefore, an urgent need exists to determine the pathogenic mechanisms of the two diseases for development of effective pharmacological therapies.

Angiotensin II (AngII) induction of AAAs is one of three commonly used mouse models of AAAs.[3] Induction of AAAs by chronic infusion of AngII was a serendipitous finding in studies that had the primary intent of determining the role of this octapeptide in hypertension-induced atherosclerosis.[4] More recently, it has been noted that AngII infusion also leads to aneurysmal formation localized to the ascending aorta.[5] Although both aneurysmal forms are induced by chronic AngII infusion, there are major distinctions in the underlying pathology of abdominal versus thoracic forms of aortic diseases.

This brief review will focus on the pathological insights in aortic aneurysms produced by AngII infusion into mice and the relevance of this model to human aortic diseases.

AngII-induced AAAs

Infusion of AngII in mice leads to rapid and progressive pathological changes in the abdominal aorta.[6,7] One aspect of similarities between AngII-induced AAAs and the human disease is the gender propensity. Like the human disease, AngII-induced AAAs exhibit marked sexual dimorphism, with males being considerable more prone to lumen expansion.[8]

The initial studies were performed in mice with gene deletion of either low-density lipoprotein receptor or apolipoprotein E that led to hypercholesterolemia. Although hypercholesterolemia has been related to development of human AAAs, the relationship is weak relative to coronary artery disease. However, subsequent studies have demonstrated that AngII-induced AAAs also occur in normocholesterolemic mice. The incidence is much less than in hypercholesterolemic mice, although there are no discernable differences in the tissue characteristics between normo- and hypercholesterolemic mice.[9]

AngII-induced AAAs exhibit highly heterogeneous pathologies. One of the most dramatic initial changes is medial rupture resulting in a grossly dilated lumen that is readily discernable by high-frequency ultrasound. A thrombus forms at the site

doi: 10.1111/j.1749-6632.2011.06332.x

of medial rupture that may also "dissect" the adventitia. These events lead to complex pathology in which a lumen dilation is adjacent to a region of intact media and remarkably expanded adventitia. Several leukocyte types migrate into the region of medial disruption, with the most prominent being macrophages and T and B lymphocytes. Continuous AngII infusion results in progressive lumen expansion and adventitial remodeling that include resolution of the thrombus.[6,7]

There are now extensive studies demonstrating the progressive and complex pathology of AngII-induced AAAs. The major emphasis of these studies has been the pathology that occurs during the initial month of AngII infusion. Within this interval, there are similarities between AngII-induced mouse AAAs and human AAA tissue including lumen expansion, extracellular matrix fragmentation, and inflammation.[6] There is progressive AAA expansion and tissue remodeling with continued AngII infusion.[7] Knowledge of the pathology of human AAAs is primarily derived from acquisition of aneurysmal tissues during open surgical repair of a profoundly dilated aorta. This is a late stage of the disease with gross distortion of tissue architecture. Unfortunately, there is a paucity of information on characteristics of human AAAs at the formative and progressive stages, while these are the disease stages that most of the animal models are probably attempting to recapitulate. Lack of fundamental knowledge of the natural history of this human disease impedes validation of these animal models.

There are two salient features of AngII-induced AAAs in mice that have the potential to differ from the human disease. One is the location of AngII-induced AAAs that contrasts the usual infrarenal location of the human disease. The development of AngII-induced AAAs in the suprarenal region has been highly consistent in all publications using this model. Interestingly, the suprarenal aorta is also the location for AAA development in other mouse models, such as mice that are hypercholesterolemic, whole body endothelial nitric oxide synthase deficiency, or smooth muscle cell-specific deficiency of low-density lipoprotein receptor-related protein.[3] The mechanistic basis for the location of AAAs is unclear in both humans and mice. One frequent inference of mechanism by which the location in the infrarenal area for human AAAs is the regional flow characteristics and changes of tissue elasticity.

Therefore, it is possible that the contrasting location during AngII infusion is due to a different location of these flow and tissue characteristics in mice versus humans.

Another commonly discussed issue is the undefined relevance of initiating processes in AngII-induced AAAs in mice to the human disease. The early event in initiation of AngII-induced AAAs is transmural medial rupture that is most commonly in the left retroperitoneal area. This occurs within days of initiating AngII infusion and forms a transmural thrombus. The initiating events in human AAAs are unknown. Although it is unlikely to be a transmural medial rupture, we speculate that a limited medial disruption could also promote thrombus formation that precipitates causal events during the evolution of human AAAs.

The causal role of the renin angiotensin system to the development of human AAAs remains to be clarified. One approach has been to determine genetic associations. One of the most commonly investigated genetic associations in the renin angiotensin system is the insertion/deletion (I/D) polymorphism of angiotensin-converting enzyme (ACE). There have been several studies to define the link between ACE I/D polymorphism and human AAAs, but these have provided conflicting results. One study has demonstrated a link between the A1166C polymorphism of the angiotensin type 1 receptor and the presence of human AAAs. This polymorphic link was replicated in datasets from three different countries. Another approach to determining the role of the renin angiotensin system in the human disease has been retrospective analysis of expansion and rupture of AAAs in patients in relation to their pharmacological treatments. Administration of ACE inhibitors has been associated with decreased rates of AAA rupture, but modest increased expansion rate. In contrast to ACE inhibitors, AngII type 1 receptor antagonists have been associated with decreased AAA expansion, while it remains unclear whether they reduce aortic rupture rate. Resolution of these conflicting findings on the association of the renin angiotensin system and AAAs will need a prospective randomized clinical trial.

A common debate is which of the three commonly used mouse models of AAAs most closely mimic mechanisms of this human aortic disease.[3] Unfortunately, we lack sufficient knowledge of the causes and natural history of human AAAs to enable assessment of the fidelity by which any of these mouse models recapitulate the human disease. The determination of pathological changes at the initiation and progression stages of human AAAs would be a major step in providing mechanistic insights and determining relevance of the mouse models. This is extremely challenging given the practical difficulties in obtaining human aortic tissues during the early phases of the disease. Conversely, the completion of double-blinded randomized trials using pharmacological inhibitors may provide the most informative approach to determining the relevance of the renin angiotensin system to the initiation, progression, and rupture of human AAAs.

AngII-induced TAAs

TAAs in humans are frequently associated with distinct genetic abnormalities that affect the integrity of the connective tissue. One of the most common is Marfan's syndrome that is caused by aberrations of the fibrillin-1 gene.[2]

In addition to the AAAs described above, AngII infusion also promotes aneurysms that are localized to the ascending aorta. However, this pathology is distinct from aneurysms that form in the abdominal aorta during AngII infusion. There is luminal expansion throughout the entire ascending aorta that progresses during prolonged AngII infusion.[7] Pathological medial changes that are present concentrically include extensive elastin fragmentation and thickening. The thickening is most profound on the adventitial aspect of the media.[5] Interestingly, the location of the AngII-induced aneurysms that form in the ascending aorta bears striking similarities to the complex distribution of embryonic origins of smooth muscle cells in the proximal aorta.

There is direct evidence that AngII has a role in the development of TAAs. Initial evidence was gleaned from a mouse model of Marfan's syndrome. Transgenic expression of one of the most common fibrillin-1 mutations in Marfan's patients (C1039G) leads to pronounced luminal expansion localized to the ascending aorta in mice. The medial architecture was also disrupted in this region. Administration of an AngII type 1 receptor antagonist, losartan, led to a complete attenuation of the aortic aneurysms. The relevance of AngII type 1 receptor antagonism has been inferred by a retrospective analysis of young Marfan's patients demonstrating that the administration of AngII type 1 receptor antagonists significantly reduced the rate of progressive aortic root expansion. There are now many ongoing double-blinded prospective studies to determine whether AngII type 1 receptor antagonism has a beneficial effect in Marfan's patients.[10]

Although there is strong evidence for a role of AngII in TAAs in patients with Marfan's syndrome, this aortic disease is also present in many non-Marfan afflicted individuals. Therefore, it will be of interest to determine the role of AngII in these diseases that are also manifested by TAAs.

Summary

AAAs and TAAs induced by AngII infusion in mice exhibit diverse pathological changes. Overall, the biggest limitation for defining the fidelity by which animal models recapitulate the pathological features of human aortic aneurysms is the deficiency in knowledge of the human diseases. This provides a strong rationale for increasing efforts in translational research of these devastating diseases.

Acknowledgment

The authors' research work is supported by Grants (HL062846 and HL80100) from the National Institutes of Health.

Conflicts of interest

The authors declare no conflict of interest.

References

1. Lederle, F.A., G.R. Johnson, S.E. Wilson, *et al.* 1997. Relationship of age, gender, race, and body size to infrarenal aortic diameter. The Aneurysm Detection and Management (ADAM) Veterans Affairs Cooperative Study Investigators. *J. Vasc. Surg.* **26:** 595–601.
2. Lindsay, M.E. & H.C. Dietz. 2011. Lessons on the pathogenesis of aneurysm from heritable conditions. *Nature* **473:** 308–316.
3. Daugherty, A. & L.A. Cassis. 2004. Mouse models of abdominal aortic aneurysms. *Arterioscler. Thromb. Vasc. Biol.* **24:** 429–434.
4. Daugherty, A., M.W. Manning & L.A. Cassis. 2000. Angiotensin II promotes atherosclerotic lesions and aneurysms in apolipoprotein E-deficient mice. *J. Clin. Invest.* **105:** 1605–1612.
5. Daugherty, A., D.L. Rateri, I.F. Charo, *et al.* 2010. Angiotensin II infusion promotes ascending aortic aneurysms: attenuation by CCR2 deficiency in apoE$^{-/-}$ mice. *Clin. Sci. (Lond.)* **118:** 681–689.
6. Saraff, K., F. Babamusta, L.A. Cassis & A. Daugherty. 2003. Aortic dissection precedes formation of aneurysms and

atherosclerosis in angiotensin II-infused, apolipoprotein E-deficient mice. *Arterioscler. Thromb. Vasc. Biol.* **23:** 1621–1626.

7. Rateri, D.L., D.A. Howatt, J.J. Moorleghen, *et al.* 2011. Prolonged infusion of angiotensin II in apoE$^{-/-}$ mice promotes macrophage recruitment with continued expansion of abdominal aortic aneurysms. *Am. J. Pathol.* **179:** 1542–1548.

8. Henriques, T.A., J. Huang, S.S. D'Souza, *et al.* 2004. Orchidectomy, but not ovariectomy, regulates angiotensin II-induced vascular diseases in apolipoprotein E-deficient mice. *Endocrinology* **145:** 3866–3872.

9. Uchida, H.A., A. Poduri, V. Subramanian, *et al.* 2011. Urokinase-type plasminogen activator deficiency in bone marrow-derived cells augments rupture of angiotensin II-induced abdominal aortic aneurysms. *Arterioscler. Thromb. Vasc. Biol.* **31:** 2845–2852.

10. Moltzer, E., J. Essers, J.H. Van Esch, *et al.* 2011. The role of the renin-angiotensin system in thoracic aortic aneurysms: clinical implications. *Pharmacol. Ther.* **131:** 50–60.

Ann. N.Y. Acad. Sci. ISSN 0077-8923

Novel, nonreflex tests detect analgesic action in rodents at clinically relevant concentrations

Nick Andrews,[1] Sinead Harper,[1] Yasmin Issop,[1] and Andrew S. C. Rice[2]

[1]Pain and Sensory Disorders Research Unit, Pfizer Laboratories, Sandwich, United Kingdom. [2]Pain Research Group, Section of Anaesthetics, Pain Medicine and Intensive Care, Faculty of Medicine, Imperial College London, London, United Kingdom

Address for correspondence: Nick Andrews, naa170767@yahoo.co.uk

We propose that predictive validity of tests for analgesia may be improved by looking to reinstate specific, innate behaviors suppressed by pain, e.g., burrowing, because effective plasma concentrations in the rat are closer to effective clinical plasma concentrations than those generally used in rodent reflex withdrawal assays.

Keywords: burrowing; chronic pain; rat

Pain influences many aspects of daily living, and effective analgesics should reinstate normal spontaneous daily behaviors. The methods historically used in laboratory animals for preclinical prediction of the efficacy of novel analgesics have recently been critically evaluated by several authors, and behavioral assessment of animals is called for.[1–3] Reflex withdrawal-based paradigms do not measure the global impact of pain *per se* and, furthermore, do not address ethological validity. Rather than trying to replicate clinical features related to human pain in the animal laboratory, predictive validity may be improved by looking to reinstate specific, innate behaviors suppressed by pain—e.g., rearing.[4] Indeed, the plasma concentrations of efficacious doses of agents with analgesic efficacy, evaluated using rearing, are in far greater agreement with effective clinical plasma concentrations than typical doses used in reflex-withdrawal based assays. For example, Matson *et al.* showed that doses as low as 3 mg/kg sc ibuprofen could reverse inflammation-induced impairments in rearing activity and this dose would be predicted to produce plasma concentrations in rats that match those seen in clinical studies.[4] Furthermore, a major advantage of looking to reinstate suppressed behaviors, rather than dampening enhanced reflexes, is that compounds that impair motor function do not seem as false positives. We have taken this philosophy forward to measure the effect of chronic pain in rats by developing a burrowing assay where levels of burrowing are reduced in rats that are in pain.[6] As with rearing, compounds or doses of compounds that impair motor activity do not seem as efficacious in this assay, but rather impair burrowing further, thus offering the user an ability to discriminate motor impairing side effects from efficacy.

Laboratory rats, *Rattus norvegicus*, are fossorial animals and, therefore, naturally burrow, unlike *Rattus rattus*, which climbs, and this behavior is highly conserved. Burrowing is extremely easy to measure objectively in laboratory rodents by weighing the amount of gravel left in the burrow at the end of the test period.[5] Burrowing is affected by a broad range of different perturbations, e.g., lesions and infections of the central nervous system as well as viral and bacterial infections, and it is suggested that the normal expression of this behavior indicates global "well being" of the rat.[5] Chronic pain can have profound effects on a patient's well-being, e.g., negative affect that leads to the patient neglecting to perform normal daily/societal tasks, such as dressing, washing, and maintaining cleanliness of the home environment or work. Therefore, measuring the effect of persistent pain on well being of the rat may offer an effective way of assessing the global effect of pain on the rat. Furthermore, by using burrowing as part of a repertoire of outcome measures for the

doi: 10.1111/j.1749-6632.2011.06342.x

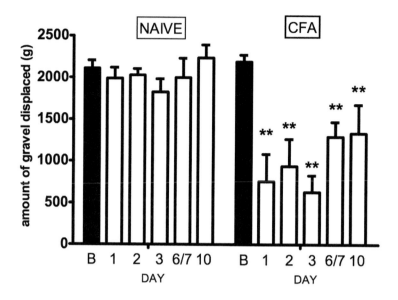

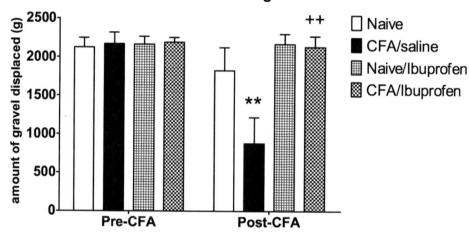

Figure 1. Upper panel shows time course of effect of CFA on burrowing over a period of 10 days. Lower panel shows effect of ibuprofen (30 mg/kg sc) on CFA-induced deficits in burrowing measured immediately before intraplantar injection of CFA and then 90 minutes postinjection of ibuprofen (three days post-CFA injection). [**] $P < 0.01$ *post hoc* test versus CFA baseline (upper panel) or naive, day 3 post-CFA (lower panel); [++]$P < 0.01$ *post hoc* test versus CFA/saline, day 3 post-CFA (lower panel).

effects of pain, the concepts of face, predictive, and construct validity may be improved.

We performed a number of studies[6] and found that the measurement of the spontaneous behavior of burrowing could be used to detect the effects of traumatic peripheral nerve injury (tibial nerve transection, L5 spinal nerve transection, and partial sciatic nerve ligation) and tissue inflammation (intraplantar Complete Freund's Adjuvant; CFA)

in the rat. The technique was simple, objective, and highly reproducible within subjects over time and was able to discriminate between a dose of a compound having specific antihyperalgesic activity and one inducing motor impairment, e.g., gabapentin 100 mg/kg i.p. reduced burrowing of rats not in pain and had no effect on the impairment of burrowing from pain, whereas gabapentin 30 mg/kg i.p. had no effect on normal burrowing but reversed the impairment of burrowing induced by peripheral nerve injury.[6] Furthermore, as with the rearing assay of Matson *et al.*[4] (see above), the clinically efficacious drugs gabapentin (30 mg/kg sc) and ibuprofen (30 mg/kg sc; Fig. 1) reversed the deficits induced by peripheral nerve injury and CFA, respectively, at doses that are lower than those generally found effective in assays using methods to evoke reflex responses. Although further work is required to understand the neurobiological and pharmacological interactions at play, we do not believe reversal of impaired burrowing by analgesics is simply an anti-stress effect, because ibuprofen, which reversed the effects of inflammation on burrowing, does not possess anxiolytic properties. Therefore, the burrowing assay described in Andrews *et al.*[6] must not be confused with the marble burying task that has been used (with little success) to detect antidepressant and anxiolytic compounds.

On the basis of these observations (see Ref. 6 for more detail), measurement of rodent behavioral activity that does not rely wholly on evoking a reflex, and crucially is ethologically relevant to the rodent, seems to deliver increased sensitivity of detection of therapeutically active analgesic compounds. With respect to the use of behaviors relevant to the rodent for assessing the impact of pain, it is possible that such approaches will be more successful than attempts to "back translate" more complex behaviors such as anxiety, depression, and cognitive effects from humans to rodents. Burrowing in particular has good face validity because pain reduces both well-being and contact-induced activity. When combined with peripheral nerve injury or inflammation, this behavior also has good construct validity.

Finally, the use of burrowing and rearing tests in rats by *in vivo* pain research scientists should enable the dissociation of selective analgesic doses of compounds from those that induce motor impairment in the same animal, thereby enabling better predictive validity (both at the level of dose and efficacy) through improved understanding of *in vivo* functional specificity.

Conflicts of interest

The authors declare no conflicts of interest.

References

1. Mogil, J.S. 2009. Animal models of pain: progress and challenges *Nat. Rev. Neurosci.* **10:** 283–294.
2. Rice, A.S.C., D. Cimino-Brown, J.C. Eisenach, *et al.* 2008. Animal models and the prediction of efficacy in clinical trials of analgesic drugs: a critical appraisal and call for uniform reporting standards. *Pain* **139:** 243–247.
3. Rice, A.S.C. 2010. Predicting analgesic efficacy from animal models of peripheral neuropathy and nerve injury: a critical view from the clinic. In *Pain 2010 An Updated Review: Refresher Course Syllabus.* J.S. Mogil, Ed.: 415–426. IASP Press. Seattle.
4. Matson, D.J., D.C. Broom, S.R. Carson, *et al.* 2007. Inflammation-induced reduction of spontaneous activity by adjuvant: a novel model to study the effect of analgesics in rats. *J. Pharmacol. Exp. Ther.* **320:** 194–201.
5. Deacon, R.M. 2006. Burrowing in rodents: a sensitive method for detecting behavioral ysfunction. *Nat. Protoc.* **1:** 118–121.
6. Andrews, N.A., E. Legg, D. Lisak, *et al.* 2011. Spontaneous burrowing behaviour in the rat is reduced by peripheral nerve injury or inflammation associated pain. *Eur. J. Pharmacol.* doi:10.1016/j.ejpain.2011.07.012.

Ann. N.Y. Acad. Sci. ISSN 0077-8923

ANNALS OF THE NEW YORK ACADEMY OF SCIENCES

Issue: *Animal Models: Their Value in Predicting Drug Efficacy and Toxicity*

Animal welfare and the 3Rs in European biomedical research

Dominic J. Wells

Department of Veterinary Basic Sciences, The Royal Veterinary College, London, United Kingdom

Address for correspondence: Dominic J. Wells, Department of Veterinary Basic Sciences, The Royal Veterinary College, London NW1 0TU, UK. dwells@rvc.ac.uk

The new Directive 2010/63/EU to ensure harmonization of animal experimentation rules has potential to increase implementation of the 3Rs (reduce, refine, replace) and improve animal welfare across Europe.

Keywords: 3Rs; animal; experimentation

Among the European countries, the United Kingdom has the longest history of regulation of the use of animals in experiments starting with legislation dating back to 1876, which introduced the requirement of personal licenses for those undertaking *in vivo* animal research and a system of inspection (an Act to amend the law relating to Cruelty to Animals, 1876). It further required that any experiment causing pain should be performed under anesthesia, that an animal should be used only once and that it should be killed at the end of the experiment.[1] This was replaced by the Animals (Scientific Procedures) Act, "A(sp)A," in 1986. This latter legislation is probably the most rigorous control of animal experiments in the world. It has further evolved over time with a series of guidance documents. A(sp)A 1986 involves a system of licensing at three levels: the institution, the project, and at the personnel level.[2] It aims to ensure animal welfare and relies on ethical judgment of costs and benefits. It is a system of national regulation via the Home Office (with political accountability) backed up by random inspections and is legally binding with a range of penalties for transgression. The associated guidance documents include details of required training and institutional ethical review.

A(sp)A is built on the concept of the 3Rs, a concept codified by Russell and Burch in 1957.[3] They argued that animal experiments should be designed to "reduce" the number of animals used to a minimum, to "refine" the way experiments are carried out to make sure animals suffer as little as possible, and wherever possible to "replace" animal experiments with nonanimal techniques. There are clear ethical reasons for carefully considering the 3Rs in animal research, but there are important economic (animal experiments are expensive) and political reasons also, as much of animal research is funded by taxpayers or charities.

Under A(sp)A 1986 there is assessment of each project on a cost-against-benefit basis, essentially asking if the ends justify the means, and aims to reduce the costs (by application of the 3Rs) and critically evaluates the likely benefits. Important questions include, "Are the studies necessary?" and "Are the experimental aims well defined and likely to yield clear answers?" Indeed, it could be argued that a second set of the 3Rs should also be considered: are the proposed experiments "relevant," "robust," and "repeatable?"

Historically, European legislation covering animal experiments varied considerably. Within the European Union (EU) member countries were required to conform to Directive 86/609/EEC. This directive required member states to adopt national legislation to "ensure that the number of animals used for experimental or other scientific purposes is reduced to a minimum, that such animals are adequately cared for, that no pain, suffering, distress, or lasting harm are inflicted unnecessarily and ensure that, where unavoidable, these shall be kept to the minimum."[4] In practice many of the member states

doi: 10.1111/j.1749-6632.2011.06335.x

Ann. N.Y. Acad. Sci. 1245 (2011) 14–16 © 2011 New York Academy of Sciences.

Table 1. A comparison of current restrictions to animal use under A(sp)A 1986 with restriction under Directive 2010/63/EU

Restrictions under A(sp)A 1986	Status under Directive 2010/63/EU
Animals may not be used for cosmetic testing.	Regulated under Directive EC 1223/2009.
Animals may not be used in developing or testing tobacco or alcohol products or offensive weapons.	No specific prohibition.
Animals may not be used for manual skills training, except microsurgery.	No specific prohibition.
No live exhibition or display of animal procedures.	No specific prohibition
No use of neuromuscular blocking agents without anesthesia.	No specific prohibition
No severe pain, distress or other suffering that cannot be controlled.	Can be allowed with specific permission from regulatory authority.
No use of Great Apes.	Can be allowed with specific permission from regulatory authority.

have effectively delegated responsibility to individual institutions, and there is wide variation in welfare standards across the EU. Directive 2010/63/EU seeks to reduce this variation between member states in terms of welfare.[5] It aims to harmonize animal research practice and legislation across Europe and appears largely based on UK A(sp)A 1986 with the same requirement for ethical justification. It entered into force on November 9, 2010 with a deadline for member states to transpose it into their legislation by November 10, 2012.

Implementation of Directive 2010/63/EU has raised a number of concerns. In the UK, there are concerns that animal welfare will be reduced by relaxation of specific constraints and changes in the regulatory process in the revision of A(sp)A 1986. It is, therefore, worthwhile comparing some of the limitations currently detailed under A(sp)A 1986 in comparison with Directive 2010/63/EU and these are listed in Table 1. Other UK groups have argued that the new Directive encourages a reduction in some of the bureaucracy that is embodied in A(sp)A 1986. In much of Europe, there are concerns over cost implications in those EU countries currently without the infrastructure that meets the new European requirements. There are also some challenges; for example, Directive 2010/63/EU requires that training/certification of competencies must be transferable between states, which is not current practice in the UK, where all prospective

licensees, even those with considerable experience, must complete some elements of mandatory training. The Federation of European Laboratory Animal Associations (FELASA) has a training scheme that fulfills part of this requirement. They have also developed guidelines for continuing professional development. However, it is likely that individual institutions will have to certify specific technical competencies. It is not yet clear how this will work across Europe.

Directive 2010/63/EU also specifically requires dissemination of best practice in animal research with particular emphasis on the 3Rs. A number of bodies such as the NC3Rs in the UK exist at national level, but it is not clear what body or bodies will be able to operate at the pan-European level. In the UK, the Home Office has recently conducted a public opinion consultation about how to implement the provisions of Directive 2010/63/EU, and it will be interesting to see how these are reflected in the revised version of A(sp)A.

In conclusion, it is clear that implementation of Directive 2010/63/EU has the potential to increase adoption of the best practice and the 3Rs across Europe and by so doing substantially increase the welfare of experimental animals. Whether this will cause some work to be transferred to other countries where regulation of animal experiments is more lax and where welfare standards may not be as high, remains to be seen.

Conflicts of interest

The author declares no conflicts of interest.

References

1. Kean, H. 2003. An exploration of the sculptures of greyfriars bobby, Edinburgh, Scotland, and the Brown Dog, Battersea, South London, England. *Soc. Animals* **1:** 353–373.

2. Animals (Scientific Procedures) Act. 1986. Her Majesty's Stationery Office UK. Pages 1–27.

3. Russell, W.M.S. & R.L. Burch. 1959. *The Principles of Humane Experimental Technique*. Methuen & Co. Ltd. London.

4. Council Directive 86/609/EEC. 1986. *Official Journal of the European Communities* **L358:** 1–28.

5. Council Directive 2010/63/EU. 2010. *Official Journal of the European Union* **L276:** 33–79.

Ann. N.Y. Acad. Sci. ISSN 0077-8923

ANNALS OF THE NEW YORK ACADEMY OF SCIENCES

Issue: *Animal Models: Their Value in Predicting Drug Efficacy and Toxicity*

Best practices for the use of animals in toxicological research and testing

William S. Stokes

National Toxicology Program Interagency Center for the Evaluation of Alternative Toxicological Methods, Division of the National Toxicology Program, National Institute of Environmental Health Sciences, National Institutes of Health, Research Triangle Park, North Carolina

Address for correspondence: William S. Stokes, D.V.M., DACLAM, Director, National Toxicology Program Interagency Center for the Evaluation of Alternative Toxicological Methods, National Institute of Environmental Health Sciences, P.O. Box 12233, Maildrop K2-16, 111 T.W. Alexander Drive, Research Triangle Park, NC 27709. Stokes@niehs.nih.gov

Animal models serve an important role in assessing preclinical safety and efficacy of new medicines and vaccines; however, such assessments can involve significant pain and distress and large numbers of animals. Best practice approaches seek to enhance animal well-being, minimize or avoid pain and distress, and use fewer animals. Advances in science and technology are providing opportunities for improved mechanism-based models and integrated safety assessments that will support improved animal welfare and reduce animal use.

Keywords: toxicology; animal welfare; animal models; alternative methods

Laboratory animal models of human disease and injury serve a vital role in translational research and testing necessary to assess the efficacy and preclinical safety of new medicines and vaccines. However, animal studies that involve development of disease or toxic injury can result in significant pain and distress, and such studies can involve large numbers of animals. Animal welfare concerns have led to national policies and laws in the United States and other countries to ensure the most humane care and use of laboratory animals and to require the consideration of alternative ways to reduce, refine, and replace animal use before studies are approved. Advances in science and technology also continue to provide new opportunities to develop improved animal models and integrated safety assessment strategies that can further reduce, refine, and replace animal use.

The concept of animal use alternatives was first described in 1959 by Rex Burch and William Russell in their book *The Principles of Humane Experimental Technique.* Commonly referred to as the "3Rs of alternatives," this concept involves *reducing* the number of animals necessary for a specific study, *replacing* animals with nonanimal systems and ap-

proaches, and *refining* animal use to enhance animal well-being or to lessen or avoid pain and distress. In the United States, the Public Health Service (PHS) Policy on Humane Care and Use of Laboratory Animals and Animal Welfare Act regulations require investigators to consider alternative methods prior to the use of animals.[1] The PHS Policy requires that studies using animals comply with the U.S. Government Principles for the Utilization and Care of Vertebrate Animals Used in Testing, Research, and Training. These principles effectively require incorporation of refinement, reduction, and replacement alternatives into animal studies to the extent that they are consistent with obtaining testing and research objectives.

NICEATM and ICCVAM

In 1993, the National Institute of Environmental Health Sciences (NIEHS), one of the National Institutes of Health, was charged by law with developing a process to achieve the regulatory acceptance of scientifically valid alternative methods that can reduce, refine, and replace animal use in testing.[2–5] In response, NIEHS established an *ad hoc* Interagency Coordinating Committee on the Validation

doi: 10.1111/j.1749-6632.2011.06334.x

of Alternative Methods (ICCVAM) to address this and other mandates. In 1997, ICCVAM was formalized as a standing committee to coordinate the interagency evaluation of the scientific validity of new, revised, and alternative methods proposed for regulatory safety testing. ICCVAM is an interagency committee consisting of 15 U.S. Federal regulatory and research agencies that use, generate, require, or disseminate safety-testing information. In the United States, Federal laws require that new safety assessment methods proposed for regulatory use must be determined to be sufficiently valid and acceptable for their intended use. ICCVAM evaluations and validation studies provide the information needed by regulatory authorities to determine if use of the proposed test method is likely to provide equivalent or improved protection of people, animals, and/or the environment.[3,5]

In 2000, the ICCVAM Authorization Act of 2000 established ICCVAM as a permanent interagency committee of the NIEHS under the National Toxicology Program Interagency Center for the Evaluation of Alternative Toxicological Methods (NICEATM) with specific purposes and duties.[6] ICCVAM and NICEATM work collaboratively to promote the validation and regulatory acceptance of new, revised, and alternative test methods based on sound science that will provide continued or improved protection of people, animals, and the environment while reducing, refining, and replacing the use of animals where scientifically feasible. NICEATM administers ICCVAM and provides scientific and technical support for ICCVAM activities. NICEATM organizes test method peer reviews and workshops in conjunction with ICCVAM and carries out independent validation studies on high priority test methods. After comprehensive scientific evaluations with multiple opportunities for public comment, ICCVAM and NICEATM forward formal recommendations to Federal agencies on test method usefulness and limitations for regulatory testing.

Since their establishment, NICEATM and ICCVAM have contributed to the evaluation of 43 alternative test methods that have been accepted or endorsed by national and international authorities. Twenty-eight of these methods are *in vitro* methods, of which most involve the use of human cells or cell lines. The other methods

involve refinement and reduction of animal-based test methods.

Animal refinement

The goals of *refinement* alternatives are to minimize or eliminate pain and distress and to enhance the well-being of animals used in research and testing. Toxicity testing often involves pain and distress because of direct or indirect tissue damage or disease resulting from the test article. Refinements not only provide for improved animal welfare, but also enhance the quality of experiments by reducing or eliminating pain and distress as an experimental variable.[1] Best practices for refinement strategies to reduce or avoid pain and distress include (1) using humane endpoints; (2) using anesthetics, analgesics, and/or tranquilizers; and (3) providing appropriate veterinary and supportive care.

Humane endpoints are criteria that can serve as the basis for ending a test procedure earlier in order to terminate or avoid pain and distress involved in the traditional study endpoint, while still allowing attainment of study objectives.[7] Humane endpoints are used to reduce the severity and/or duration of pain and distress experienced by an animal.[7] Clinical signs, physiologic parameters, biochemical measurements, and other parameters can serve as potential earlier biomarkers of humane endpoints. Humane endpoints are especially useful when medications cannot be used to treat pain and distress, due to interference of the medications with study objectives. The ideal humane endpoints are those that can be used as criteria to end a procedure *before* the onset of animal pain and distress.[7]

Humane endpoints have been developed to reduce animal pain and distress associated with potency testing of vaccines, where a challenge test with live pathogens is required. For example, earlier humane endpoints for veterinary rabies vaccines have been approved and adopted for use in the United States and internationally.[8] The onset of paresis, paralysis, and/or convulsions was determined to sufficiently predict rabies infection and indicate that the animal would not recover. Use of these humane endpoints results in euthanasia of animals two to three days before death would normally occur.

The local lymph node assay (LLNA) is an example of an alternative test method where use of an earlier mechanistic humane endpoint completely avoids the pain and distress previously involved in traditional tests used to determine the allergic contact dermatitis potential of chemicals.[2,7,8] The traditional test method, using either the Buehler or the guinea pig maximization test, requires observation for actual elicitation of allergic dermatitis, which is manifest by redness, swelling, and pruritis. In contrast, the LLNA uses an earlier, more sensitive biomarker that avoids the need to evoke the potentially painful elicitation phase of the traditional methods. The LLNA measures changes to one of the key biological pathway events required for the development of chemically-induced allergic contact dermatitis (ACD), namely, lymphocyte proliferation in the lymph nodes that drain the skin area where the test article is applied repeatedly. The LLNA only assesses events that occur during the induction phase of ACD and therefore avoids the need for exposure from a later chemical challenge necessary to elicit an allergic response. Other advantages of the LLNA are that it uses at least 40% fewer animals, involves a much shorter time to perform, and does not require the use of potentially irritating adjuvants commonly used in the traditional guinea pig test.[3,7]

Anesthetics and analgesics can be used to reduce or avoid pain and distress in certain test situations. For example, ICCVAM recently recommended that pain management procedures should always be used in animal studies that are necessary to determine the eye injury potential of test substances.[2,8] These preemptive procedures include the routine use of topical anesthetics and systemic analgesics prior to the application of test articles to the eye. Systemic analgesics are then continued until eye lesions resolve or the study is terminated. Frequent evaluation and recording of eye injuries is also conducted throughout the study, including observation for clinical signs and lesions that can serve as humane endpoints to terminate the study early.

Appropriate veterinary and supportive care is essential for assuring animal well-being and should always be provided to minimize discomfort in animals used in testing and research studies. This includes frequent observation of animals to identify clinical signs and the provision of care necessary to reduce or alleviate pain and distress, or to address injuries or other adverse effects. Appropriate interventions should be made to allow the animals to maintain good hydration, to obtain necessary access to food, and to have a clean and dry environment.

Animal reduction

Reduction alternatives are approaches and methods that result in attainment of study objectives with fewer animals. The up-and-down procedure (UDP) is an example of how animal use for assessing acute oral toxicity has been reduced by at least 80% with an innovative statistical approach and sequential animal testing.[3,4] The traditional LD_{50} (median lethal dose) test used as many as 200 animals per test, while the UDP typically only uses three to seven animals per test. Since acute oral toxicity is the most commonly conducted safety test worldwide, this alternative test method has profoundly reduced animal use for regulatory safety testing more than any other single test.

Integrated decision strategies that incorporate *in vitro* test methods are increasingly being used in an integrated approach to assess the safety or potential toxicity of various chemicals, medicines, and products.[4] Integrated decision strategies use multiple sources of data and information and can increase the certainty of hazard and safety predictions beyond the certainty associated with only a single source of data or information. Such approaches can also reduce animal use and reduce uncertainties in extrapolating from animals to humans.

Animal replacement

Replacement alternatives are those that use nonanimal methods—such as cell, tissue, and organ cultures—or nonsentient phylogenetically lower species, such as insects. Animal models have been largely replaced for many testing situations, such as the replacement of rabbits for endotoxin testing by the bacterial endotoxin and human monocyte activation tests.[2,5] A recent example of a replacement alternative is an engineered cell line approved by the U.S. Food and Drug Administration as a substitute for the mouse LD_{50} potency test for release of botulinum therapeutic products.

Future progress

In recent years there has been a growing emphasis on developing and using *systems biology* approaches to understand how early chemical perturbations of genetic and cellular functional pathways can lead to adverse health outcomes. These approaches include a wide range of tools that incorporate toxicogenomics, metabolomics, proteomics, cell-based assays, biochemical activity profiles, and computational models. Information from these tools is used to create biological activity profiles, with an expectation that such profiles will eventually predict toxicity or safety and eliminate the need to observe actual adverse outcomes in animal models.[8,9] The development of systems biology approaches has been stimulated by advances in new technologies and an enhanced understanding of the molecular and cellular mechanisms of toxicity. These tools are also helping to identify more sensitive and earlier biomarkers of toxicity that will likely be incorporated into future *in vitro* and animal safety testing methods.

NIEHS and the National Toxicity Program (NTP) support basic and applied research that may lead to development of new test methods relevant to regulatory testing. These include the Tox 21 collaboration between the NTP, the NIH Chemical Genomics Center, FDA, and the U.S. Environmental Protection Agency.[8,10] The Tox 21 initiative is the largest *in vitro* toxicology research program ever conducted worldwide and is expected to yield candidate methods and approaches with potential applicability to regulatory testing. Following standardization and validation in consultation with ICCVAM, methods with regulatory applicability will be reviewed by ICCVAM and recommendations forwarded to appropriate agencies.

Summary

Best practices for the use of animals in research and testing involves consideration and use of innovative methods and approaches that can enhance animal well-being, minimize or avoid pain and distress, and reduce the number of animals required to obtain scientifically valid results. The continued application of new science and technology to develop and validate scientifically sound models and earlier humane endpoints is expected to further improve animal welfare and further reduce and replace animal use, while ensuring and advancing the health of people, animals, and the environment.

Conflicts of interest

The author declares no conflicts of interest.

References

1. Stokes, W.S. 1997. Animal use alternatives in research and testing: obligation and opportunity. *Lab. Animal* **26**: 28–32.
2. ICCVAM. 2010. ICCVAM Biennial Progress Report 2008–2009, NIH Publication No. 10-7612, NIEHS, Research Triangle Park, NC, USA, October 2008. Available at: http://iccvam.niehs.nih.gov/about/ICCVAMrpts.htm.
3. Stokes, W.S. & L.M. Schechtman. 2007. Validation and regulatory acceptance of new, revised, and alternative toxicological methods. In *Principles and Methods of Toxicology*. A.W. Hayes, Ed.: 1103–1128. Taylor and Francis. Philadelphia, Pennsylvania.
4. Stokes, W.S. & M. Wind. 2010. Recent progress and future directions at NICEATM-ICCVAM: validation and regulatory acceptance of alternative test methods that reduce, refine, and replace animal use. *ALTEX* **27**: 221–232.
5. Birnbaum, L. & W. Stokes. 2010. Safety testing: moving toward alternative methods. *Environ. Health Perspect.* **118**: A12–A13.
6. ICCVAM Authorization Act. 2000. 42 U.S.C. 2000. Public Law 106–545.
7. Stokes, W.S. 2002. Humane endpoints for laboratory animals used in regulatory testing. *ILAR J.* **43**: S31–S38.
8. Stokes, W.S. & M. Wind. 2010. Validation of innovative technologies and strategies for regulatory safety assessment methods: challenges and opportunities. *ALTEX* **27**: 87–95.
9. NRC. 2007. *Toxicity Testing in the 21st Century: A Vision and a Strategy*. National Academies Press. Washington, DC.
10. Collins, F.S., G.M. Gray & J.R. Bucher. 2008. Toxicology. Transforming environmental health protection. *Science* **319**: 906–907.

Ann. N.Y. Acad. Sci. ISSN 0077-8923

ANNALS OF THE NEW YORK ACADEMY OF SCIENCES
Issue: *Animal Models: Their Value in Predicting Drug Efficacy and Toxicity*

Progress toward generating informative porcine biomedical models using induced pluripotent stem cells

Franklin West and Steven Stice

ADS Department, University of Georgia Regenerative Bioscience Center, University of Georgia, Athens, Georgia

Address for correspondence: Steven Stice, 425 River Rd., ADS Rhodes Complex, University of Georgia, Athens, GA 30602. sstice@uga.edu

Porcine induced pluripotent stem cells hold significant promise in modeling human biomedical regenerative medicine and as translational large animal disease models.

Keywords: pig; induced pluripotent; stem cells

Informative, complex, gene-targeted murine biomedical models are possible, in part, because pluripotent stem cells enable multiple gene modifications and selection, and germline transmission of traits. Complex and repeated gene targeting for porcine biomedical models would compliment rodent models if robust porcine stem cells become available. In addition, porcine pluripotent stem cells could be used to model human allogenic stem cell regenerative therapeutics in a large animal model (the pig) and for preclinical large animal testing of therapeutic compounds at a fraction of the cost of nonhuman primate studies. The promise and utility of porcine-induced pluripotent stem (piPS) cells are directly linked to their pluripotent stem cell characteristics: infinite expansion, clonal isolation, differentiating into any cell type in the body *in vitro* and *in vivo*, and incorporation into the germline of chimeric animals.[1–5] These characteristics enable the knock-in or knock-out of multiple genes, the production of homogeneous populations of altered cells, and the development of cell lines and animals that have desired characteristics not previously obtainable in any species outside of the mouse.

The need to robustly produce highly genetically engineered biomedical pigs is obvious. Pig models for a number of diseases, such as atherosclerosis to cystic fibrosis, are likely to be superior to their rodent counterparts. Cystic fibrosis patients typically have abnormal paranasal sinus development and lung disease characterized by chronic airway infec-

tions and inflammation.[6,7] However, this does not occur in mouse models, which makes it impossible to study the molecular causes of these symptoms in mice. The pig is a likely model because it is similar in size to humans and has a longer lifespan than mice, which enables researchers to conduct more extensive and long-term studies of disease progression with age. Because pig and human organ size and physiology are in many respects similar, the pig is considered the most probable source of cells and organs for xenotransplantation. Overexpression of human genes, such as decay-accelerating factor, CD46, and CD59, and the knockout of α-1,3-galactosyltransferase in donor pigs has significantly improved pig-to-primate transplantation by preventing immune rejection.[8,9] However, xenotransplanted tissues still fail to thrive for more than a few months even when these factors are overexpressed or removed, suggesting that more extensive gene modifications will be required to overcome the complex immune responses stimulated by xenotransplantation. In both pig disease and xenotransplant models, the addition or removal of multiple genes will be likely necessary to produce animals similar enough to humans and to use pig models to their full potential.

Our research team has recently generated piPS cells that show morphology, immunoreactivity, and *in vitro* differentiation characteristics indicative of a pluripotent state (Table 1).[2,3] However, previous attempts to make pluripotent embryonic stem cells

doi: 10.1111/j.1749-6632.2011.06337.x

Table 1. Established Pluripotency Characteristics of Pig Induced Pluripotent Stem Cells

High nucleus/ cytoplasm ratio	Large nucleoli	AP	EB	Teratomas	Chimeras	References
Yes	Yes	High	Yes; formed all three germ layers	–	Yes; germline	2, 3
Yes	Yes	High	Yes; formed all three germ layers	Yes; formed all three germ layers	–	4
Yes	Yes	High	–	Yes; formed all three germ layers	–	5
Yes	Yes	High	Yes; formed all three germ layers	Yes; formed all three germ layers	–	1

(ESCs) from pigs have demonstrated that cells can be generated that have ESC character but are unable to produce chimeric animals—the most stringent and definitive test of pluripotency. Thus, these cells were not truly pluripotent.

To test the pluripotency of piPS cells, 10–15 cells were introduced into blastocyst stage embryos and transferred to recipient animals.[3] Piglets produced from these embryos were tested at fetal and post-parturition stages of development for the presence of exogenous POU5F1 and NANOG genes (used in the piPS cell reprogramming process) to determine if piPS cells had successfully incorporated into the developing blastocyst. Testing for pluripotency *in vivo* in this way generated animals that were highly chimeric and demonstrated that piPS cells were capable of contributing to all three germ layers and, ultimately, the germline.[3] These findings showed that piPS cells can reach a fully reprogrammed state from which they can participate in the formation of germline chimeric animals.

In addition, in a recent publication, we addressed the concern that piPS cells may continue to express reprogramming factors and have an altered reprogrammed epigenome that leads to changed function and/or teratomas in chimeric animals.[3] Our results showed that piPS cells, although contributing to chimeric animals, did not alter the phenotype of these individuals. This may indicate that iPS cells in nonmurine species are more easily tolerated and less likely to generate teratomas, reinforcing the goal of generating comparative and complimentary large and small animal models for disease and cell therapies.

Despite significant advances, piPS cells produced by several groups have shown significant variability.[1–5] The heterogeneity of the reprogramming process, leading to diverse levels of pluripotency gene and protein expression, high epigenetic variability, and ultimately significant divergence in plasticity between iPS cell lines, is a potential contributing factor to the variability seen. Further studies addressing the overall goal of understanding genetic and epigenetic contributions to porcine reprogramming will potentially enhance the potency of nonmurine stem cells. Ultimately, for use of piPS cells to be successful and for piPS cells to reach their full potential, these cells must maintain their pluripotency through extended gene modification and culture, and then contribute to the germline of chimeric pigs.

An alternate approach is to use genetically modified iPS cells with nuclear transfer to generate offspring without the need to generate germline chimeras. Efficient and limited gene targeting is possible with somatic cell nuclear transfer, which avoids the need to have pluripotent cells for less complex modifications. However, as gene modifications become more complex, somatic cells may senesce over time in culture. Combining piPS cells that are immortal with nuclear transfer avoids the issue of cells senescing before completion of adding or modifying all genes of interest. Porcine iPS cells will likely be used in far-reaching applications, and combined with existing gene modification and methods, they will ultimately help generate informative and valuable large animal models, resources, and cell sources for therapeutic applications.

Conflicts of interest

The authors declare no conflicts of interest.

References

1. Ezashi, T. *et al*. 2009. Derivation of induced pluripotent stem cells from pig somatic cells. *Proc. Natl. Acad. Sci. U.S.A.* **106:** 10993–10998.
2. West, F.D. *et al*. 2010. Porcine induced pluripotent stem cells produce chimeric offspring. *Stem. Cells Dev.* **19:** 1211–1220.
3. West, F.D. *et al*. 2011. Chimeric Pigs produced from induced pluripotent stem cells demonstrate germline transmission and no evidence of tumor formation in young Pigs. *Stem. Cells* **29:** 1640–1643.
4. Wu, Z. *et al*. 2009. Generation of Pig-induced pluripotent stem cells with a drug-inducible system. *J. Mol. Cell Biol.* **1:** 46–54.
5. Esteban, M.A. *et al*. 2009. Generation of induced pluripotent stem cell lines from Tibetan miniature pig. *J. Biol. Chem.* **284:** 17634–17640.
6. Rogers, C.S. *et al*. 2008. Disruption of the CFTR gene produces a model of cystic fibrosis in newborn pigs. *Science* **321:** 1837–1841.
7. Ostedgaard, L.S. *et al*. 2011. The DeltaF508 mutation causes CFTR misprocessing and cystic fibrosis-like disease in pigs. *Sci. Transl. Med.* **74:** 1–24.
8. Byrne, G.W. *et al*. 1997. Transgenic pigs expressing human CD59 and decay-accelerating factor produce an intrinsic barrier to complement-mediated damage. *Transplantation* **63:** 149–155.
9. Cooper, D.K. *et al*. 1993. Identification of alpha-galactosyl and other carbohydrate epitopes that are bound by human anti-pig antibodies: relevance to discordant xenografting in man. *Transpl. Immunol.* **3:** 198–205.

Ann. N.Y. Acad. Sci. ISSN 0077-8923

ANNALS OF THE NEW YORK ACADEMY OF SCIENCES

Issue: *Animal Models: Their Value in Predicting Drug Efficacy and Toxicity*

A knockout mouse resource for the biomedical research community

K. C. Kent Lloyd

Mouse Biology Program, University of California Davis, Davis, California

Address for correspondence: K. C. Kent Lloyd, Mouse Biology Program, University of California, 2795 Second Street, Suite 400, Davis, CA 95618. kclloyd@ucdavis.edu

The Knockout Mouse Project (KOMP) Repository archives and distributes vectors, embryonic stem cell clones, frozen germplasm, and live mutant mice for 8,500 knockout genes. Here, we describe the creation and functions of the KOMP Repository.

Keywords: genetically altered mice; knockouts; gene targeting; ES cells

Since its inception in the mid-1980s, gene targeting by homologous recombination in mouse embryonic stem (ES) cells has transformed the ability to functionally assess individual genes in mice for the study of systems biology in health and disease.[1] Just a few years ago, the National Institutes of Health (NIH) discovered that after awarding hundreds of millions of dollars over two decades to individual laboratories, large and small, only ~4,000 unique mouse strains had been generated, and even fewer, 700 or so, were publicly available without restriction. In response, and to capitalize on newly sequenced whole genomes, improvements in construct and vector design, and technological advances in gene targeting and ES cells, a recently coordinated program[2] involving projects in the United States[3] and Europe[4] has used unconventional high-throughput approaches to derive a comprehensive library of ES cells with loss-of-function alleles, covering nearly every protein-coding gene in the mouse genome.[5] The close homology between the mouse and human genomes[6] and the promise for identifying genetic factors in mice that may inform human disease pathogenesis is a compelling rationale for converting the entire ES cell resource into mice. Further, these facts provide convincing evidence for the scientific value of a concerted effort to strategically analyze the resultant knockout mouse resource.

To extend the benefit of these large-scale efforts to knockout the entire mouse genome to the world-wide community of biomedical researchers, repositories have been created to archive and distribute the newly generated materials and data, and to make them available and accessible to any and every scientist. One of these repositories is made up of a consortium between the University of California Davis (UCD) and Children's Hospital Oakland Research Institute (CHORI), which serves as the repository for all products generated in the NIH Knockout Mouse Project (KOMP) Mutagenesis Program. As the lead institution, UCD archives, maintains, conducts quality assurance, and fulfills orders for ES cell clones, live mouse lines, and frozen embryos and sperm, whereas CHORI fulfills similar requests for targeting vectors. The repository ensures the viability, genotype, pathogen-free status, and chromosome count of all KOMP products.

To date, the repository has imported 75,302 targeted ES cell clones for 6,909 unique genes from the two teams (CHORI–Sanger–UCD Consortium and Regeneron, Inc.) participating in the KOMP Mutagenesis Program. After quality assurance testing, 70,754 ES cell clones for 6,503 genes have been made available for ordering and distribution. Eventually, products for 8,500 knockout targeted genes, most conditional ready, will be available. Since initial operations began four years ago, the repository has fulfilled 2,770 (84%) of 3,316 orders received for ES cell clones, doing so by aiming to respond to orders within 8–12 weeks of a request. The repository now

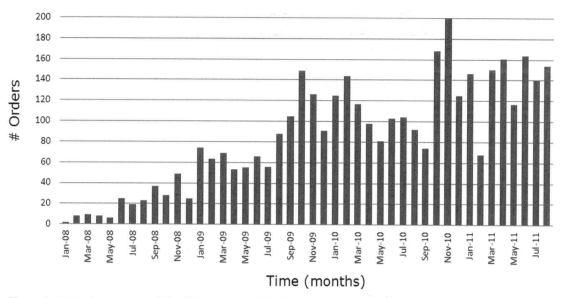

Figure 1. Orders for gene-targeted ES cell clones generated by the KOMP Mutagenesis Program and archived and distributed by the KOMP Repository. The steady increase in orders (average ∼150/month over the last six to nine months) from the global research community demonstrates the scientific value and promise of this resource to facilitate the study of the genetic basis of disease.

receives and fulfills on average of more than 150 orders per month for vectors, ES cell clones, and mice (Fig. 1). Most investigators use KOMP ES cells and/or chimeras obtained from the KOMP Repository to generate mutant mouse colonies to use for hypothesis-driven scientific study.

The repository also provides valuable services, such as microinjection, to convert ES cells to mice. To date, the repository has injected 938 unique clones into either BALB/c or B6D2F1 × C57BL/6 host blastocysts to produce chimeras for germline transmission testing. Of 659 clones for which testcrosses have been completed, 446 (68%) successfully transmitted through the germline. These data suggest that injection of three clones per gene will ensure a >96% likelihood (1–[0.32 × 0.32 × 0.32]) of achieving germline transmission. All KOMP Repository products and services are available to both academic and commercial entities for a modest cost. Because the NIH intended the resource to become self-sustaining, fees charged to obtain KOMP products are used to ensure continued maintenance and operation of the repository. Special pricing packages are available to reduce costs to researchers. For example, instead of purchasing an individual ES cell clone for US$648, a customer can save by purchasing a "premium ES cell package" for US$2,801, which includes up to three in-

jectable clones per gene and guaranteed quality control assurance, including growth and viability testing, genotyping confirmation, pathogen screening, and chromosome count. Alternatively, investigators can purchase a premium microinjection service for US$10,691, which guarantees production of at least one >50% male chimera or there is no charge. By creating a *my*KOMP account and registering interest in specific KOMP genes, investigators will be sent email notification announcing that products on their interest list are available and can be ordered from the repository. To date, more than 6,000 scientists from around the world have created accounts and expressed interest in over 3,200 genes.

In an effort to seek feedback on the scientific utility of KOMP products, the repository conducts surveys of their researcher clients and requests feedback on their success using KOMP ES cells. For example, in response to an email questionnaire to 524 investigators who had ordered 454 clones, 209 (42%) respondents reported that 227 (83%) of 273 clones injected in their labs had resulted in the birth of chimeras. Of these, 117 (63%) of 185 clones that have completed germline transmission testing had been successful. In another survey of 70 customers who had ordered microinjection and delivery of chimeras, 52 (74%) reported that 34 (71%) of 48 clones that produced chimeras had successfully transmitted through the germline. Once completed, NIH-funded investigators can fulfill their obligations under the NIH Sharing Policy by depositing into the repository mice made in their laboratory from KOMP products. Under the KOMP Sharing Plan, researchers who return at least two germline-confirmed, heterozygous KOMP mutant male mice on a congenic C57BL/6N genetic background within one year of purchase of ES cell clones and/or chimeras will receive an immediate cash refund of 50% the cost of purchasing ES cells or US$1,000 refund of the cost of microinjection. Mutant mice sent to the KOMP Repository and passing stringent quality assurance procedures are made available for distribution to other investigators and are cryopreserved as frozen germplasm for safety, security, and distribution.

The repository maintains an easily navigable website (www.komp.org) where users can search, browse, and order products and services from the online catalog. In addition, users can access and download protocols, contact customer and technical services (1–888-KOMP-MICE, service@komp.org), read news updates, follow the KOMP blog, view FAQs, and more. Besides ensuring the utility, longevity, and vitality of this unique resource, the KOMP Repository is key to the success of KOMP-Phase 2, which seeks to conduct comprehensive, high-throughput phenotypic screening to functionally annotate all protein-coding genes in the mammalian genome.[7]

Conflicts of interest

The author declares no conflicts of interest.

References

1. van der Weyden, L., D.J. Adams & A. Bradley. 2002. Tools for targeted manipulation of the mouse genome. *Physiol. Genomics* **11:** 133–164.
2. Collins, F.S., J. Rossant & W.A. Wurst. 2007. A mouse for all reasons: the international mouse knockout consortium. *Cell* **128:** 9–13.
3. Austin, C.P. *et al.* 2004. The knockout mouse project. *Nat. Genet.* **36:** 921–924.
4. Auwerx, J. *et al.* 2004. The European dimension for the mouse genome mutagenesis program. *Nat. Genet.* **36:** 925–927.
5. Skarnes, W.C. *et al.* 2011. A conditional knockout resource for the genome-wide study of mouse gene function. *Nature* **474:** 337–344.
6. Waterston, R.H. *et al.* 2002. Initial sequencing and comparative analysis of the mouse genome. *Nature* **420:** 520–562.
7. Abbott, A. 2010. Mouse project to find each gene's role, international mouse phenotyping consortium launches with a massive funding commitment. *Nature* **465:** 410.

Ann. N.Y. Acad. Sci. ISSN 0077-8923

ANNALS OF THE NEW YORK ACADEMY OF SCIENCES

Issue: *Animal Models: Their Value in Predicting Drug Efficacy and Toxicity*

Minimizing strain influences in a genetically modified mouse phenotyping platform

Michael D. Hayward, Olesia Buiakova, and David S. Grass

Taconic, Discovery & Preclinical Research Solutions, Cranbury, New Jersey

Address for correspondence: Michael D. Hayward, Ph.D., Taconic, 5 Cedar Brook Drive, Cranbury, NJ 08512.
Michael.Hayward@Taconic.com

Our approach has been to power studies to allow for detection of at least modest changes from a wild-type littermate control, include assays with overlapping physiological systems to provide cross-functional interpretive value, and to employ challenge assays.

Keywords: mice; phenotyping; disease models

Few issues have generated more cynicism about the use of genetically modified mouse models (GEMs) in research than the influence of genetic background on a primary phenotypic characterization. The different strains (and substrains) of mice can be a problematic source of variability in data generated by studies of genetic modifications in mice maintained on multiple background strains. Commonly, problems arise by mixing different strains during the generation of genetically modified founder lines, especially when complex inducible mutations are introduced, and in subsequent breeding schemes. An improvement in genetic homogeneity has been offered by the availability of C57BL/6 (B6) embryonic stem (ES) cells and the use of albino B6 or BALB/c mice as recipients to screen for likely germline-positive founders. However, the large availability of lines that have already been created on mixed backgrounds reduces the incentive to re-create lines on congenic strains. In addition, there has been a failure to appreciate the existence of multiple substrains of inbred strains of mice with the possible exception of the many 129 substrains and the ES cells derived from those different substrains.[1] Thus, recently we have been reliving that experience with the several B6 substrains that exist. Finally, the creation of congenic lines has to take into consideration the phenotypes of the inbred line itself, where some physiological systems may differ widely among the different sub-

strains and be at odds with human physiology. For these reasons, we have attempted to minimize the influence of strains in our commercial phenotyping platform by using an approach that maximizes the chances of detecting relevant phenotypes.

Heterogeneity of strain genetic backgrounds is a common concern in characterizing genetically modified mice. Genetic modifications created in the germ line can result in phenotypes whose identification is limited to certain inbred strains (for an example, see Ref. 2). In addition, baseline responses of inbred mice can vary in many established assays. Examples of this include the *disc1* mutation in many of the 129 strains that leads to impaired performance in some cognition assays.[3] Genetic heterogeneity created by mixing background strains can confound data interpretation, resulting in the identification of phenotypes mistakenly assumed to be related to the genetic modification when they are actually related to the features of the parental inbred strain(s). The mixing of backgrounds also frequently leads to increased standard deviation (i.e., "noise") in the data, possibly masking statistically significant results.

Although the contribution of the genetic background of mouse strains has been appreciated, and even exploited in quantitative trait loci studies, the genetic effects of different substrains has not been appreciated to nearly the same degree. The

doi: 10.1111/j.1749-6632.2011.06333.x

backcrossing of GEMs to 129 substrains was noted as being more complicated due to the large number and genetic diversity of 129 substrains some years ago.[1] Recently, with the more common use of B6 ES cells and breeding to congenicity on the B6 background, it is increasingly recognized that there exist differing substrains of B6 mice with clear genetic diversity among these substrains. Most notable is the *Nnt* null mutation that exists in the C57BL6J substrain but not in other substrains, such as C57BL6N and C57BL6JBom.[4] In fact, our studies have revealed divergence between the C57BL/6J and C57BL/6NTac substrains in body weight and glucohomeostasis when challenged on a high fat diet.[5] Additional studies have revealed differences in baseline responses to nociception, cognition, and anxiety.[6,7]

Despite the complications created by the diversity of inbred mouse lines, there are ways of minimizing its effects in the design of studies on GEMs. The most optimal solution is to generate a targeted mutation in an ES cell line that is isogenic to the line to be bred to. However, in many cases this solution is not available, due to high economic demand or due to inability to identify a specific phenotype on certain genetic backgrounds.

We designed a pragmatic approach to phenotyping a large number of mouse lines with varying degrees of mixed backgrounds. The principles that went into this design include:

(1) breed heterozygotes to produce littermates for the study;
(2) understand assay characteristics and relevant magnitude of effect; use power calculations to help balance breeding costs and the level of sensitivity in an assay;
(3) To minimize breeding costs, conduct multiple assays on the same mice using a strategic and validated design; and
(4) use synonymous assays to confirm phenotypes.

One general principle, therefore, was to use a study group size that was appropriate for the given assay and statistical power inherent to that assay, as predicted from the standard deviation of the results from mice on a similar background (mixed or inbred). For example, behavioral assays used 10–25 mice per group and nonbehavioral assays used 5–10

mice per group. To be the most efficient with breeding costs, both sexes were used but, in most cases, only one sex was used for each assay. We also designed the platform with cross-validation of assays by including functionally (but not technically) related assays. For example, the formalin assay and the hot plate assay were both used for baseline nociception, dual X-ray absorptiometry (DEXA) and μCT for adipose composition, and elevated plus maze and open field for anxiety-related behaviors. We also included assays that probe overlapping physiology *in vivo* with complimentary *ex vivo* assays. For example, we tested glucose tolerance *in vivo* and serum adiponectin levels *ex vivo* for insulin sensitivity, DEXA scan *in vivo* and serum leptin levels *ex vivo* for obesity, tail-bleeding test *in vivo*, and *ex vivo* coagulation for blood coagulation. Finally, we included challenge assays, for example, a high-fat diet challenge, which allows for normalizing data to initial baseline measurements, which helps to decrease standard deviations.

Our comprehensive phenotyping platform employed for the evaluation of genetic targets pioneered the approach of using a fully validated panel of assays conducted in series (Fig. 1). This decreases the time line to characterize the requested knockout (KO) line by minimizing breeding time lines. This platform is currently marketed as "PhenoTac." PhenoTac is a fully validated panel of assays conducted serially (i.e., multiplexing assays), where the placement of each assay within the protocol was validated by comparing the results to naive mice. The comprehensive platform allows for the identification of unpredicted phenotypes, which in our experience, have been detected in nearly half of all KO lines that we have characterized. The serial design ensures that a majority of the resources go toward characterizing the mice in assays, rather than for breeding mice in preparation for subsequent phenotypic characterization (Fig. 1).

A good understanding of the nature of the assay, and how it can be applied to a phenotyping study, is particularly important and frequently overlooked. A power analysis employed on mice of differing genetic backgrounds provides an appropriately powered study design. Inherent in such an analysis is an understanding of the biological and clinical relevance of the sensitivity of an assay. Small differences in an assay can be highly meaningful, such as blood pressure in mice, whereas only a large

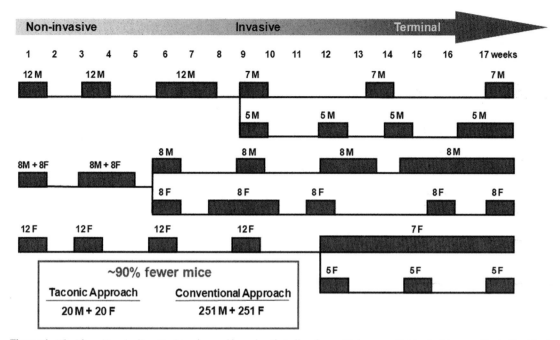

Figure 1. The PhenoTac pipeline consists of several branches that allow for multiple sequential *in vivo* bioassays (including bleeds for multiple measurements) on a defined cohort of mice. In this example, 29 assays were performed on cohorts of 40 KO mice and 40 wild-type mice. Each block represents an individual assay; the number above the block gives the group size (*N*) and sex of the group being tested. If the same assays were conducted on individual groups of mice, a total of 502 KO and 502 wild-type mice would be required.

difference in other assays is meaningful, such as pre-pulse inhibition.

The diversity inherent among the inbred strains can also be exploited by breeding for particular phenotypes to be used as animal models of human diseases. One could argue that without the existence of the many inbred strains, many of the mouse models of human diseases would not even exist. For example, the DIO model gained its present recognition in obesity and diabetes research because C57BL/6 substrains, unlike some other mouse strains, are susceptible to obesity and prediabetic phenotypes (hyperglycemia and insulin resistance) induced by a calorically dense diet. Another example is an Alzheimer disease model generated by introducing a mutated amyloid peptide precursor gene (*Swe* mutation) into wild-type mice. The mutation is described on several different genetic backgrounds and its phenotypic manifestation varies depending on the background. On 129S6 and on a mixed background of B6;SJL, mice with the *Swe* mutation show cognitive deficits and morphological and biochemical changes in the brain that parallel findings in Alzheimer patients. However, other backgrounds do

not even support the long-term survival of mice carrying this transgene. This diversity among inbred strains can also be used to determine how critical the contribution of a particular gene to a certain phenotype is, by comparing the gene mutation penetrance on different backgrounds. For example, the reduced motivation (by mice) to bar press for palatable food reinforcers by enkephalin KO mice was measured on two different backgrounds, C57BL/6J and DBA/2J, while a knockout of the β-endorphin peptide only reduced the motivation when on a C57BL/6J background.[2] Thus, while the existence of different strains (and substrains) of mice have complicated breeding and assay design, different strains have also been exploited to develop better animal models.

There are many disease models that are strain specific—highlighting the importance of understanding the effects of strain background on the model. In this short overview, we discussed several strategies to minimize unwanted influence of background strain on studies that are aimed at characterizing genetically modified mice. The choice of ES cells and the breeding strategies employed are fundamental to a study design meant to reduce the influence of multiple strains on identification of phenotypes. With a carefully designed strategy, the use of genetically modified mice can provide important information that is not practical by alternative methods. The existence of the differing strains of mice can also be employed in disease models that are strain specific.

Conflicts of interest

All authors are employees of Taconic.

References

1. Simpson, E.M., C.C. Linder, E.E. Sargent, *et al.* 1997. Genetic variation among 129 substrains and its importance for targeted mutagenesis in mice. *Nat. Genet.* **16**: 19–27.
2. Hayward, M.D., A. Schaich-Borg, J.E. Pintar & M.J. Low. 2006. Differential involvement of endogenous opioids in sucrose consumption and food reinforcement. *Pharmacol. Biochem. Behav.* **85**: 601–611.
3. Clapcote, S.J. & J.C. Roder. 2006. Deletion polymorphism of Disc1 is common to all 129 mouse substrains: implications for gene-targeting studies of brain function. *Genetics* **173**: 2407–2410.
4. Mekada, K., K. Abe, A. Murakami, *et al.* 2009. Genetic differences among C57BL/6 substrains. *Exp. Anim.* **58**: 141–149.
5. Hayward, M.D., T. Chu, S. Karagrigoriou, *et al.* 2011. A Comparison of Metabolic Characteristics Among C57BL/6NTac, C57BL/6J and C57BL/6JBom Diet Induced Obese Mice With Environmental Conditioning. In: *Book A Comparison of Metabolic Characteristics Among C57BL/6NTac, C57BL/6J and C57BL/6JBom Diet Induced Obese Mice With Environmental Conditioning.* Abstract #P3-372. The Endocrine Society's 93rd Annual Meeting and Expo; Boston.
6. Bryant, C.D., N.N. Zhang, G. Sokoloff, *et al.* 2008. Behavioral differences among C57BL/6 substrains: implications for transgenic and knockout studies. *J. Neurogenet.* **22**: 315–331.
7. Matsuo, N., K. Takao, K. Nakanishi, *et al.* 2010. Behavioral profiles of three C57BL/6 substrains. *Front. Behav. Neurosci.* **4**: 29.

Ann. N.Y. Acad. Sci. ISSN 0077-8923

ANNALS OF THE NEW YORK ACADEMY OF SCIENCES
Issue: *Animal Models: Their Value in Predicting Drug Efficacy and Toxicity*

The blessings and curses of C57BL/6 substrains in mouse genetic studies

Camron D. Bryant

Department of Human Genetics, The University of Chicago, Chicago, Illinois

Address for correspondence: Camron D. Bryant, Ph.D., Department of Human Genetics, The University of Chicago, 920 E. 58th St., CLSC 501, Chicago, IL 60637. camron@uchicago.edu

Phenotypic and genetic differences among C57BL/6 substrains are accumulating. Investigators must address these differences to improve the quality of their studies.

Keywords: B6; inbred; KOMP; next-generation sequencing; QTL mapping

The C57BL/6 (B6) mouse strain is the most widely used strain in biomedical research, with nearly 25,000 articles on Pubmed documenting its use. Nearly half of these articles cite the use of C57BL/6J (B6/J), the original B6 strain from the Jackson Laboratory (JAX) from which all other B6 substrains were derived. In 1951, the first B6 substrain, C57BL/6N (B6/N), was created after breeders were shipped to the National Institutes of Health. Hundreds of generations later, a number of genetic and phenotypic differences have been reported between B6/J and B6/N. This paper discusses how these differences arose, the problems of treating B6 substrains as equals, and our present state of knowledge regarding these differences. I will also outline specific action items for dealing with the unavoidable use of multiple B6 substrains in genetic engineering studies and opportunities that B6 substrains offer for finding novel genes contributing to complex traits.

Theoretically, the essence of an inbred strain is that each individual shares the same homozygous allele for every DNA sequence in the genome and thus, is genetically identical. Furthermore, a common assumption is that this fixation is genetically stable across time. In reality, a very small amount of the genome between any two individuals will always differ, owing in part to unique residual heterozygosity that averted fixation during inbreeding and spontaneous mutations that introduce *de novo* het-

erozygosity. These genomic impurities can eventually become fixed and lead to the formation of a new substrain. This fixation occurs more rapidly when a small number of founders are used to establish a new B6 colony and could quickly contribute to deviation in one's favorite phenotype and, thus, to the creation of a new substrain.

The B6 inbred strain is a popular choice for researchers conducting behavioral studies because it is physically active, capable of learning a variety of tasks, and breeds frequently. Furthermore, phenotypic differences among B6 substrains (sometimes very large differences) can offer flexibility in studying many behaviors. Behavioral differences between B6/J and B6/N in ethanol consumption and preference were noted in the early 1980s and have since been replicated in at least two laboratories (reviewed in Bryant *et al.*[1]). Other examples of large, replicable phenotypic differences between B6/J and B6/N include fear learning and anxiety that is greater in B6/N than in B6/J, whereas pain sensitivity and rotarod performance are greater in B6/J than in B6/N.[1,2] These differences allow investigators to choose the most appropriate B6 substrain for their experiments. For example, because the B6/J strain readily drinks ethanol, this strain is appropriate for examining manipulations that are hypothesized to decrease ethanol consumption. In addition, because the B6/N strain shows a large degree of fear learning, this strain is the most appropriate choice for

doi: 10.1111/j.1749-6632.2011.06325.x

studying manipulations expected to decrease fear. The advantage of choosing among B6 substrains as opposed to other inbred strains is that the results might be more applicable for reverse genetic studies (e.g., knockouts and transgenics), which overwhelmingly use B6 mice. However, investigators do not always report the specific substrain employed, making it difficult to know which one is appropriate for a particular phenotype.

The Knockout Mouse Project (KOMP) is an international effort to create mice harboring null mutations for each protein-coding gene in the mouse genome.[3] The B6/N strain was employed as the choice of embryonic stem (ES) cell line for harboring these mutations, likely because of its technical superiority over B6/J.[4] However, the specific B6/N substrain used for KOMP is not entirely clear. Before the advent of KOMP, a majority of genetic engineering studies used ES cells from a substrain of 129 origin to harbor the mutation, mainly because of the high success rate of germline transmission following blastocyst injection. The use of B6/N offers two perceived advantages. First, there is no longer any need to backcross mutant mice to B6 to create a congenic mouse with an isogenic background—this is both expensive and time consuming. Second, the criticism that polymorphisms in the congenic region that flanked the mutation could cause the phenotype[5] is no longer valid. However, unless the exact same B6 substrain is used to introduce the mutation, and to backcross, there still is cause for concern that a mixed background or the congenic region could account for the results.

In examining a recent large dataset providing SNPs among B6 substrains, there are approximately 150 SNPs with homozygous calls that distinguish B6/J from B6/N, depending on the specific substrain comparison. In contrast, the N substrains seem to be much more similar to each other, differing at only 10–20 homozygous SNPs out of several hundred thousand.[6] Recently published next-generation sequencing data of C57BL/6J and C57BL/6NJ (an N substrain that is now bred at JAX) from the Wellcome Trust Center at the Sanger Institute reveal much more potential genetic variation.[7,8] Even when just considering nonsynonymous coding SNPs, there are more than 80 high-confidence SNP calls and over 400 putative ones. In addition, there are thousands of other

SNPs that could affect transcript and splice variant levels and structural or copy number variants. A query for this dataset is provided by the Wellcome Trust at http://www.sanger.ac.uk/cgi-bin/modelorgs/mousegenomes/snps.pl. It is clear that the genetic differences between B6/J and B6/N are quite extensive and most likely contribute to phenotypic variation. Thus, if a KOMP-generated mutation (B6/N derived) is placed on a B6/J background, the same problems that were thought to be overcome with B6/N ES cells still exist: the phenotypic effect of the KOMP mutation could depend on the mixed B6/J and B6/N backgrounds or the effect thought to be caused by the KOMP mutation could actually be caused by an N/J genetic variant that is in linkage disequilibrium with the null mutation on a congenic background.

As the list of variants distinguishing B6 substrains continues to grow, what action should investigators take to address the potential problems that can be anticipated from using a B6 background strain that is different from the KOMP B6/N strain? First and foremost, there is a need to carefully document which substrains are used for ES cell generation and backcrossing and to treat these substrains as different strains, not as equal ones. Second, it would be extremely helpful for those investigators who suspect that their previous findings might be explained by B6 substrain differences to address this possibility and to report any revised conclusions.[9] Furthermore, the choice of B6 background strain for a genetic engineering study should be tailored to the specific phenotype. If a B6/J strain must be used as the background, sequencing the congenic boundary flanking the transgene and comparing these results with the latest sequencing data will define how many polymorphic genes within the congenic region could potentially affect the phenotype.

Although genetic differences among B6 substrains present problems for reverse genetic studies, these same differences offer opportunities for forward genetic studies, which thrive on genetic and phenotypic variation. The identification of genomic regions harboring B6 variants associated with variance in a trait (quantitative trait loci [QTL]) could rapidly lead to the identification of genes harboring the genetic variants. Because the genetic backgrounds between any two B6 substrains are nearly identical, the majority of the genome can be eliminated in considering which genes underlie the QTLs. The usefulness of this approach for B6 substrains has yet to be tested and will depend on both the amount and distribution of genetic variation that underlies a QTL. If the SNPs are highly abundant and widely distributed across most of the genes, then the typical problems of F2 studies will still exist: low resolution and hundreds of genes to parse among. If however, the SNPs are limited to a finite number of genes, then it might be possible to narrow the gene list to a sizeable number of candidates. A recent study using C57BL/6J and the closely related C57L/J and C58/J strains suggest that this approach will be useful.[10]

To summarize, researchers must beware of the differences among B6 substrains if their contribution to forward and reverse genetic approaches to complex traits is to be fully realized. If researchers are prepared to address these differences, they can minimize their potential confounding effects and, at the same time, maximize the chance for novel gene discovery. It will be important to sequence the genomes of other substrains of B6/J and B6/N because behavioral and genetic differences exist even within strains derived from each of these two core substrains.[1] Finally, it is important to consider that environmental differences may also play an important role in phenotypic variation among B6 substrains and, thus, this question can be addressed by cross-fostering studies and other approaches that attempt to control for the substrain environment.

Conflicts of interest

The author declares no conflicts of interest.

References

1. Bryant, C.D., N.N. Zhang, G. Sokoloff, *et al.* 2008. Behavioral differences among C57BL/6 substrains: implications for transgenic and knockout studies. *J. Neurogenet.* **22:** 315–331.
2. Matsuo, N., K. Takao, K. Nakanishi, *et al.* 2010. Behavioral profiles of three C57BL/6 substrains. *Front. Behav. Neurosci.* **4:** 1–12.
3. Austin, C.P., J.F. Battey, A. Bradley, *et al.* 2004. The knockout mouse project. *Nat. Genet.* **36:** 921–924.
4. Pettitt, S.J., Q. Liang, X.Y. Rairdan, *et al.* 2009. Agouti C57BL/6N embryonic stem cells for mouse genetic resources. *Nat. Methods.* **6:** 493–495.
5. Gerlai, R. 1996. Gene-targeting studies of mammalian behavior: is it the mutation or the background genotype? *Trends. Neurosci.* **19:** 177–181.
6. Yang, H., J.R. Wang, J.P. Didion & R.J. Buus. 2011. Subspecific origin and haplotype diversity in the laboratory mouse. *Nat. Genet.* **43:** 648–655.
7. Keane, T.M., L. Goodstadt, P. Danecek, *et al.* 2011. Mouse genomic variation and its effect on phenotypes and gene regulation. *Nature.* **477:** 289–294.
8. Yalcin, B., K. Wong, A. Agam, *et al.* 2011. Sequence-based characterization of structural variation in the mouse genome. *Nature.* **477:** 326–329.
9. Bourdi, M., J.S. Davies & L.R. Pohl. 2011. Mispairing C57BL/6 substrains of genetically engineered mice and wild-type controls can lead to confounding results as it did in studies of JNK2 in acetaminophen and concanavalin A liver injury. *Chem. Res. Toxicol.* **24:** 794–796.
10. Eisener-Dorman, A.F., L. Grabowski-Boase, B.M. Steffy, *et al.* 2010. Quantitative trait locus and haplotype mapping in closely related inbred strains identifies a locus for open field behavior. *Mamm. Genome.* **21:** 231–246.

Ann. N.Y. Acad. Sci. ISSN 0077-8923

ANNALS OF THE NEW YORK ACADEMY OF SCIENCES

Issue: *Animal Models: Their Value in Predicting Drug Efficacy and Toxicity*

Modeling inflammation and microvascular dysfunction

Felicity N.E. Gavins

Imperial College London, London, United Kingdom

Address for correspondence: Felicity N. E. Gavins, Imperial College London, Wolfson Neuroscience Laboratories, Imperial College Faculty of Medicine, Hammersmith Hospital Campus, Burlington Danes Building, Du Cane Road, London W12 0NN, UK. f.gavins@imperial.ac.uk

We are using confocal intravital microscopy to understand the mechanisms behind leukocyte trafficking in the brain, thus providing potential therapeutic targets for neurovascular diseases, for example, stroke and multiple sclerosis.

Keywords: inflammation; microvasculature; dysfunction

Under normal circumstances, the body is capable of restoring homeostasis following insults due to a variety of pathogens and noxious stimuli that enter the system. Injury that occurs to the human body provokes a typical "host response" of pain, fever, redness, swelling, and loss of function. These classical signs are collectively referred to as "inflammation," and in some cases, excessive and/or prolonged inflammation can lead to extensive tissue damage, organ dysfunction, and mortality, which are associated with a number of different diseases including myocardial infarction, stroke, and sepsis.

The microcirculation is highly responsive to, and a vital participant in, the inflammatory response. All segments of the microvasculature, i.e., arterioles, capillaries, and venules, are affected by, and contribute to, the inflammatory response.[1] The inflammatory response is characterized by an infiltration of leukocytes (monocytes, neutrophils, and eosinophils), the major cellular defense mechanism. This leukocyte infiltration is achieved by a complex interaction between selectins and integrins in response to chemoattractants such as complement factors, leukotriene B4, and platelet-activating factor. This inflammatory process involves a number of intricate and complex steps, including leukocyte capture (or tethering), slow rolling, adhesion strengthening and spreading, intravascular crawling, and transmigration (either via a transcellular (through endothelial cells) or a paracellular (be-

tween endothelial cells) route into the site of tissue injury.[2]

Significant research effort has been directed toward understanding the mechanisms that initiate and regulate the inflammatory response in disease. A number of imaging techniques have been employed to help quantify these mechanisms, such as the specialized technique of intravital microscopy (IVM). Certainly, the main advantage of using imaging for drug discovery is achieved by the ability of high-resolution microscopic imaging to measure spatial and temporal distribution of molecules and cellular components, which is vital to understanding the activity of drug targets, biomarkers, and drug effect at the cellular level.

IVM is an innovative technique that provides quantitative, *in-vivo* real-time imaging of cellular interactions (such as leukocyte–endothelial cell interaction), thus offering a cost-effective approach to accelerate preclinical development. It enables the user to gain insight into molecular (e.g., pharmacokinetics and promoter activity), cellular (e.g., leukocyte-endothelial cell interactions), and anatomical (e.g., vascular architecture and pore size) areas.[3]

My group, and others, have used this technique to understand not only normal physiology, but also the pathophysiology of human disease. In particular, we have been interested in understanding the mechanism of a variety of anti-inflammatory drug targets that may cause the resolution of the inflammatory

doi: 10.1111/j.1749-6632.2011.06344.x

Ann. N.Y. Acad. Sci. 1245 (2011) 34–35 © 2011 New York Academy of Sciences.

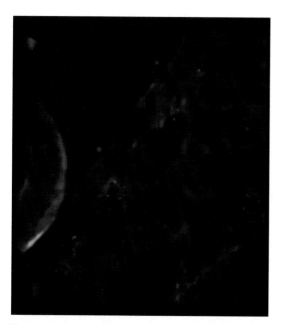

Figure 1. Inflamed murine cerebral vessel. Ischaemia was induced in the murine brain by occlusion of the middle cerebral artery, followed by a period of reperfusion. Confocal intravital microscopy was employed to visualize leukocyte interactions with the endothelium. Cerebral vessels were immunostained *in vivo* for endothelial cell junctions by IV injection of FITC labeled Ab to PECAM-1 (green), neutrophils were labeled with Rhodamine mAb to CD45.2 (red), and leukocytes were labeled with Cy5 mAb to Gr-1 (blue). Original magnification, 40×.

three-dimensional observation of leukocyte transmigration in real-time (four-dimensional imaging) pre- and poststroke. As such, this technique allows for critical examination of the mechanisms by which leukocytes cross cerebral vessel walls, something that is currently unknown, and thus may provide potential therapeutic targets for a number of neurovascular diseases, such as stroke and multiple sclerosis (both of which share an inflammatory component). Evidence of the complexities of leukocyte transmigration in other vascular beds using this technique have shown that different adhesion molecules mediate the effects, and these appear to be stimulus specific.[8] Whether the same can be said for the brain remains to be seen.

These are indeed exciting times for those studying the inflammatory process and leukocyte trafficking. The use of more sophisticated dyes/fluorescent markers and the availability of a wide variety of genetically manipulated animals, combined with the use of confocal IVM, will help to better understand the complex role of the leukocyte.

Conflicts of interest

The author declares no conflicts of interest.

References

1. Vacharajani, V. & D.N. Granger. 2009. Adipose tissue: a motor for the inflammation associated with obesity. *IUBMB Life* **61:** 424–430.
2. Ley, K. *et al.* 2007. Getting to the site of inflammation: the leukocyte adhesion cascade updated. *Nat. Rev. Immunol.* **7:** 678–689.
3. Hughes, E.L. & F.N. Gavins. 2010. Troubleshooting methods: using intravital microscopy in drug research. *J. Pharmacol. Toxicol. Methods* **61:** 102–112.
4. Gavins, F.N. 2010. Are formyl peptide receptors novel targets for therapeutic intervention in ischaemia-reperfusion injury? *Trends Pharmacol. Sci.* **31:** 266–276.
5. Perretti, M. *et al.* 1996. Mobilizing lipocortin 1 in adherent human leukocytes downregulates their transmigration. *Nat. Med.* **2:** 1259–1262.
6. Ye, R.D. *et al.* 2009. International union of basic and clinical pharmacology. LXXIII. Nomenclature for the formyl peptide receptor (FPR) family. *Pharmacol. Rev.* **61:** 119–161.
7. Gavins, F.N. *et al.* 2007. Activation of the annexin 1 counter-regulatory circuit affords protection in the mouse brain microcirculation. *FASEB J.* **21:** 1751–1758.
8. Voisin, M.B., D. Pröbstl & S. Nourshargh. 2010. Venular basement membranes ubiquitously express matrix protein low-expression regions: characterization in multiple tissues and remodeling during inflammation. *Am. J. Pathol.* **176:** 482–495.

process in different diseases.[4] One particular compound of interest is the anti-inflammatory protein annexin 1,[5] which we have demonstrated, with the use of IVM, to cause leukocyte detachment from the endothelium in different vascular beds (e.g., cremaster, mesentery, and brain).[6] Of particular interest, we (and other groups) have shown that the effect of annexin 1 is mediated by the formyl peptide receptor (FPR) family.[6,7]

Our main area of research focuses on ischemia reperfusion (I/R) injury, which is a common feature of several diseases associated with high morbidity and mortality, such as stroke and myocardial infarction.[4] Growing evidence suggests that members of the FPR family, in particular human FPR2/ALX, may have an important role in the pathophysiology of I/R injury. We are currently studying this in the context of I/R in the brain.[7] In particular, we are now using confocal IVM to understand cell trafficking and thus the inflammatory response in the brain (Fig. 1). The highly specialized technique enables

Ann. N.Y. Acad. Sci. ISSN 0077-8923

ANNALS OF THE NEW YORK ACADEMY OF SCIENCES
Issue: *Animal Models: Their Value in Predicting Drug Efficacy and Toxicity*

TRPV1 and TRPA1 channels in inflammatory pain: elucidating mechanisms

Susan D. Brain

BHF Centre of Cardiovascular Excellence and Section of Integrative Biomedicine, King's College London, London, United Kingdom

Address for correspondence: Susan D. Brain, Cardiovascular Division and Section of Integrative Biomedicine, King's College London, Franklin-Wilkins Building, Waterloo Campus, London SE1 9NH, UK. sue.brain@kcl.ac.uk

Transient receptor potential (TRP) receptors are ion channels that mediate pain and inflammation. We provide evidence for the distinct roles of TRPV1 and TRPA1 in arthritis.

Keywords: hyperalgesia; pain; TRP channels; mice

Transient receptor potential (TRP) receptors are thermo-sensing, ligand-gated, nonselective cation channels that mediate pain and inflammation. We and others have presented evidence for the role of TRP vanilloid 1 (TRPV1) channels in arthritis. We now have evidence that the colocalized TRP ankyrin 1 (TRPA1) channels are also involved in pain processing in a chronic murine CFA-induced monoarthritis model, albeit by distinct mechanisms compared to TRPV1.

Pain associated with rheumatoid arthritis can be severe and difficult to control. Alternatively, although the pain may not be severe, it can have a disabling and depressing influence, and it is a common reason for the patient to seek referral to specialist treatment units, incurring loss of work and high medical costs. The common pain relief agents that are heavily prescribed are associated with limitations. The objective of our research is to work at a fundamental level to learn more about the role of sensory nerves and their receptors in inflammatory hyperalgesia/allodynia. Our ultimate aim is to provide mechanistic evidence for feasible and relevant novel therapeutic targets for arthritis. We have evidence that TRPA1 may be such a target and have evaluated mechanisms by which it may act to enhance pain and inflammatory mechanisms in arthritis.

Sensory nerves consisting of C and Aδ fibers innervate joints and skin and are often located in close association with blood vessels. Sensory afferents terminate in and around the joint, the stimulation of nerves in the inflamed joints is considered to play a primary role in arthritic pain, and their antidromic stimulation leads to release of neuropeptides, with increased joint blood flow and edema formation.[1] Our earlier research focused on the neuropeptides substance P and, more specifically, CGRP, which are released from stimulated sensory nerves in rats. More recently, we have additionally studied murine models of inflammatory hyperalgesia. This has led us to investigate bilateral thermal and mechanical hyperalgesia pain responses in the mouse.[2–4] Symmetrical pain hypersensitivity implies the involvement of a neuronal pathway and, indeed, hyperexcitability of nociceptive pathways.

It is now realized that certain members of the TRP receptors are key molecular integrators of the initiation and maintenance of joint pain, although the precise mechanisms responsible for these activities are unclear.[5] We previously investigated the role of TRPV1 in the mediation of bilateral thermal and mechanical hyperalgesia, pain modalities associated with inflammatory hyperalgesia.[2,4] We demonstrated that deletion of TRPV1 is important for mediating thermal hyperalgesia and inflammatory swelling after CFA-induced joint inflammation.[2] This study was supported by other complementary studies, with some also showing that the severity of arthritis in rodent models was reduced when TRPV1 was either blocked or deleted. Capsaicin creams, which stimulate and then desensitize sensory nerves and act via the TRPV1 receptor,[5] have been shown to benefit osteoarthritis,

doi: 10.1111/j.1749-6632.2011.06326.x

but are associated with a burning sensation. More recently, TRPV1 antagonists have been developed, and evidence from rodent models indicates a beneficial effect of such agents in reducing arthritic pain, although an adverse effect of hyperthermia is delaying translation to human disease studies.

The TRPA1 channel is like TRPV1, a nonselective cation channel. Evidence suggests that it is expressed in a proportion, approximately 30–50%, of TRPV1, containing sensory neurons.[6] TRPA1 is activated by a distinct range of stimulants, including plant irritants such as mustard oil (allyl isothyocyanate), cinnamon (cinnamaldehyde), and thymol. Of greater endogenous importance, reactive oxygen species and their peroxidation metabolites are also known as TRPA1 agonists. The TRPA1 receptor responds to temperature changes of $<17\,^{\circ}$C *in vitro*[7] and, depending on circumstances, is sensitive to cold *in vivo*.[8]

It is known that TNF-α levels in joint exudate remain high in the absence of TRPV1 in CFA-induced monoarthritis.[2] The success of anti-TNF-α antibodies in arthritis treatment indicates that TNF-α plays a primary pathophysiological role in arthritis. Anti-TNF-α biologicals also alleviate arthritic pain in humans, in addition to slowing disease progression, although it is unclear how TNF-α mediates inflammatory pain.

We recently focused on TNF-α–mediated thermal hyperalgesia as a model and demonstrated that it is linked to a series of peripheral events—involving TRPV1, COX-2–dependent prostaglandins, and IL-1β—that maintains thermal hyperalgesia.[3] More recently, we examined mechanisms involved in TNF-α–induced mechanical hyperalgesia and demonstrated, with the use of TRPA1 antagonists and TRPA1 knockout (KO) mice, a clear involvement of TRPA1.[4] Two selective TRPA1 receptor antagonists, HC-030031 and AP-18, inhibit mechanical hyperalgesia mediated by CFA.[9,10] We have confirmed and extended results with AP-18 to show an analgesic effect on secondary hyperalgesia when AP-18 is injected into the murine knee joint with established CFA-induced monoarthritis. Furthermore, we have now examined the TRPA1-dependent mechanisms involved in mechanical hyperalgesia observed in a chronic model of CFA-induced monoarthritis. Experiments with wild type and TRPA1-KO mice over four weeks revealed a peripheral involvement of TRPA1 in maintaining mechanical hyperalgesia induced by CFA.[4] These findings support the hypothesis that although TRPA1 may not be involved in the acute inflammatory pain observed after CFA, it plays a critical role in maintaining the inflammatory pain over two to three weeks after induction of monojoint arthritis.

Thus, our work has reached a stage where we have novel evidence that TRPA1 may influence inflammatory pain in a distinct manner to that already known for TRPV1. This raises the possibility that TRPA1 antagonists in addition to TRPV1 antagonists play a role and moreover that a dual antagonist may also be beneficial through blockade of the distinct TRPA1/V1 mechanisms.

Conflicts of interest

The author declares no conflicts of interest.

References

1. Ferrell, W.R. & N.J. Russell. 1986. Extravasation in the knee induced by antidromic stimulation of articular C fibre afferents of the anaesthetized cat. *J. Physiol.* **379:** 407–416.
2. Keeble, J., F. Russell, B. Curtis, *et al.* 2005. Involvement of transient receptor potential vanilloid 1 in the vascular and hyperalgesic components of joint inflammation. *Arthritis. Rheum.* **52:** 3248–3256.
3. Russell, F.A., E.S. Fernandes, J.P. Courade, *et al.* 2009. Tumour necrosis factor alpha mediates transient receptor potential vanilloid 1-dependent bilateral thermal hyperalgesia with distinct peripheral roles of interleukin-1beta, protein kinase C and cyclooxygenase-2 signalling. *Pain.* **142:** 264–274.
4. Fernandes, E., F. Russell, R. Graepel, *et al.* 2011. A distinct role for TRPA1, in addition to TRPV1, in mechanical hypernociception induced by TNFα and in CFA-induced monoarthritis. *Arthritis. Rheum.* **63:** 819–829.
5. Szallasi, A., F. Cruz & P. Geppetti. 2006. TRPV1: a therapeutic target for novel analgesic drugs? *Trends. Mol. Med.* **12:** 545–554.
6. Kobayashi, K., T. Fukuoka, K. Obata, *et al.* 2005. Distinct expression of TRPM8, TRPA1, and TRPV1 mRNAs in rat primary afferent neurons with adelta/c-fibers and colocalization with trk receptors. *J. Comp. Neurol.* **493:** 596–606.
7. Story, G.M., A.M. Peier, A.J. Reeve, *et al.* 2003. ANKTM1: a TRP-like channel expressed in nociceptive neurons, is activated by cold temperatures. *Cell.* **112:** 819–829.
8. Kwan, K.Y. & D.P. Corey. 2009. Burning cold: involvement of TRPA1 in noxious cold sensation. *J. Gen. Physiol.* **133:** 251–256.
9. Petrus, M., A.M. Peier, M. Bandell, *et al.* 2007. A role of TRPA1 in mechanical hyperalgesia is revealed by pharmacological inhibition. *Mol. Pain.* 17;3:40.
10. Eid, S.R., E.D. Crown, E.L. Moore, *et al.* 2008. HC-030031, a TRPA1 selective antagonist, attenuates inflammatory- and neuropathy-induced mechanical hypersensitivity. *Mol. Pain.* **4:** 48.

Ann. N.Y. Acad. Sci. ISSN 0077-8923

ANNALS OF THE NEW YORK ACADEMY OF SCIENCES

Issue: *Animal Models: Their Value in Predicting Drug Efficacy and Toxicity*

Imaging of endocrine gene expression in a humanized transgenic rat

Julian R.E. Davis

University of Manchester, Manchester, United Kingdom

Address for correspondence: Julian R.E. Davis, University of Manchester, Manchester M13 9PT, United Kingdom.
julian.davis@manchester.ac.uk

Reporter gene imaging has revealed cyclical patterns of gene expression in living cells. Transgenic animal studies show that these patterns are modified by tissue architecture.

Keywords: gene regulation; cell imaging; pituitary; prolactin

Huge advances have been made in our understanding of gene regulation using traditional biochemical techniques that rely on DNA and protein extracts from tissues and cells. In the last few years however, the use of bioluminescent and fluorescent reporter genes has led to the discovery that gene promoter activity in individual living cells is highly variable and fluctuates over the course of hours.

We have studied the regulation of the pituitary hormone gene, prolactin, an important reproductive hormone in humans and mammals, and the product of the commonest form of pituitary tumor in man. Reporter genes have been used for many years to understand gene promoter structure and function and the role of different transcription factors and coactivator and repressor proteins. Firefly luciferase and destabilized green fluorescent protein (d2EGFP) are reporter genes with short half-lives, which has enabled their use as surrogate markers of transcription rate. Mathematical modeling to take account of their slightly different mRNA and protein half-lives can generate directly comparable estimates of transcription rate.[1]

Using cell lines we have found that prolactin gene expression is highly variable from hour to hour,[2] and autocorrelation function analysis has shown that most cells display a dominant cycle periodicity of approximately 10 hours. This cyclical gene expression is therefore not a circadian phenomenon nor related to cell cycle, and evidence so far suggests that this phenomenon is because of cycles of chromatin remodeling.[3]

Studies in cell lines have major limitations, however: pituitary GH3 cells are aneuploid, lack receptors for important hypothalamic regulatory factors such as dopamine, and display continued proliferation in culture, unlike the mostly postmitotic cells of the normal pituitary gland. We have therefore taken a transgenic approach to allow us to study cycles of gene expression in normal cells and tissues. Rats have the important advantage over mice for this particular application that a small endocrine gland can be more readily studied *in vivo* because of the larger size of the animal, and in addition, endocrine physiology is better understood in the rat than the mouse. We generated recombinant bacterial artificial chromosomes (BACs) to encompass a large fragment (160 kbp) of the human prolactin gene locus.[4] The human gene locus differs substantially from the rodent locus in that it contains an alternate distant promoter that confers differential regulation on the gene in different tissues in humans and primates.[5] The recombinant BAC approach therefore enables studies that closely resemble the "authentic" regulation of a given locus in a series of tissues and physiological circumstances that would not otherwise be accessible in humans.

Imaging of the intact living animal confirmed the expected expression of the transgene in the pituitary gland but also indicated that after

doi: 10.1111/j.1749-6632.2011.06341.x

inflammatory stress the transgene was activated in various nonpituitary tissues, including the peritoneal cavity, where transgene activation was found to be because of infiltrating monocytes/macrophages (Ref. 4 and preliminary data).

The expression of the transgene in the pituitary gland was studied in more detail comparing dispersed cell preparations to "intact" tissue preparations using a tissue slice approach as has been developed by other groups.[6] Using this approach, we found that the structure of the intact pituitary gland constrains patterns of gene expression so that they are more coordinated and synchronized.[7] Furthermore, studies of the fetal pituitary gland showed that as nascent pituitary endocrine cells start to differentiate and first express their hormone gene, they display marked cycles of expression, and these become stabilized as neighboring cells start to form contiguous cell networks in postnatal life.[8]

The ability to study animal models has therefore allowed the translation of basic molecular biological insights into tissue physiology and has started to illustrate how tissue architecture has important effects on the patterns of gene expression *in vivo*. In addition, the transgenic approach allows investigators to study tissue specific patterns of gene expression that reflect the evolution of human gene loci in ways that would not be replicated by the endogenous rodent genes. In the case of prolactin, this has given us important insights into the potential role of prolactin as a proinflammatory cytokine and has illustrated potential new therapeutic targets in inflammatory responses. The translation of novel applications of bioluminescent and fluorescent reporter proteins[9] to understand physiological regulation is leading to important new insights in *in vivo* mammalian biology.

Acknowledgments

This work was supported by program grants to J.R.E.D., M.R.H. White (University of Manchester), J.J. Mullins (University of Edinburgh), and D.A. Rand (University of Warwick) from the Wellcome Trust, UK.

Conflicts of interest

The author declares no conflicts of interest.

References

1. Finkenstädt, B., E.A. Heron, M. Komorowski, *et al.* 2008. Reconstruction of transcriptional dynamics from gene reporter data using differential equations. *Bioinformatics* **24:** 2901–2907.
2. Takasuka, N., M.R.H. White, W.R. Robertson & J.R.E. Davis. 1998. Dynamic changes in prolactin promoter activation in individual living lactotrophic cells. *Endocrinology* **139:** 1361–1368.
3. Harper, C.V., B. Finkenstädt, D. Woodcock, *et al.* 2011. Long-term unsynchronised transcriptional cycles individual living mammalian cells. *PLoS Biol.* **9:** 1000607, 1–14.
4. Semprini, S., S. Friedrichsen, C.V. Harper, *et al.* 2009. Real-time visualisation of human prolactin alternate promoter usage *in vivo* using a double-transgenic rat model. *Mol. Endocrinol.* **23:** 529–538.
5. Gerlo, S., J.R.E. Davis, D. Mager & R. Kooijman. 2006. Primate prolactin: a tale of two promoters. *BioEssays* **28:** 1051–1055.
6. Bonnefont, X., A. Lacampagne, A. Sanchez-Hormigo, *et al.* 2005. Revealing the large-scale network organization of growth hormone-secreting cells. *Proc. Natl. Acad. Sci. U.S.A.* **102:** 16880–16885.
7. Harper, CV., K. Featherstone, K. Semprini, *et al.* 2010. Dynamic organization of prolactin gene expression in living pituitary tissue. *J. Cell Sci.* **123:** 424–430.
8. Featherstone, K., C.V. Harper, A. McNamara, *et al.* 2011. Pulsatile patterns of pituitary hormone gene expression change during development. *J. Cell Sci.* **124:** 3484–3491.
9. Spiller, D.G., C.D. Wood, D.A. Rand & M.R.H. White. 2010. Measurement of single cell dynamics. *Nature* **465:** 736–745.

Ann. N.Y. Acad. Sci. ISSN 0077-8923

ANNALS OF THE NEW YORK ACADEMY OF SCIENCES

Issue: *Animal Models: Their Value in Predicting Drug Efficacy and Toxicity*

Systems biology of the heart: hype or hope?

T. Alexander Quinn[1,2] and Peter Kohl[1,2]

[1]National Heart and Lung Institute, Imperial College London, London, United Kingdom. [2]Department of Computer Science, University of Oxford, Oxford, United Kingdom

Address for correspondence: T. Alexander Quinn, Cardiac Biophysics and Systems Biology Group, National Heart and Lung Institute, Imperial College London, Heart Science Centre, Harefield UB9 6JH, UK. t.quinn@imperial.ac.uk

Systems biology, the approach that combines reduction and integration to explore dynamic structure–function interrelations across biomedically relevant spatio-temporal scales, is applied to heart research.

Keywords: model; cardiac structure; cardiac function

Whether one subscribes to the view that *systems biology* is a field of study, a set of techniques, or a conceptual approach, it has become a mainstream element of biomedical research. Although there seems to be no universally acceptable definition for the term yet, the smallest common denominator is perhaps that systems biology considers the *mutual interactions between a biological entity and its parts*.[1] This can be derived directly from the definitions of *biology* (contracted from *bios* [Greek for "life"] and *logos* [Greek for "word, study"]: "the study of life") and *system* (according to Ludwig von Bertalanffy, "an entity that maintains its existence through the mutual interaction of its parts").[2]

Systems biology, whether targeting the level of populations, whole organisms, organs, tissues, cells, or subcellular components, builds on a combination of experimental, theoretical, and computational techniques. These are applied, from the outset, with the aim to support both "reductionist" (attempting to understanding the nature of complex systems by reducing them to the interactions of their parts) and "integrationist" (focusing on systems-level properties and how those shape lower level behavior) approaches for studying the dynamic interplay of biological structure and function within the biological system of interest. This synthesis of formerly disparate (and, at least apparently, opposing) approaches to biomedical research requires novel concepts and tools, in particular for tackling the challenge associated with conducting research that requires investigation at multiple levels of structural complexity (e.g., study how cells, integrated into tis-

sues, support organ function). Another interesting aspect is that parts of a system at one level (e.g., cells in a muscle) constitute systems in their own right at a lower level of structural complexity (e.g., for the investigation of calcium handling effects on cross-bridge formation).[3]

Biological research, whether aiming primarily to reduce or to integrate, relies on *models*. By definition, models *are simplified representations of reality*.

This definition applies to all models, whether conceptual, experimental, or computational. As the extent and scope of simplification will differ between models, there is no one-to-one map between "reality" and "model." Thus, if we are interested in the effects of pharmacological modulation of one ion channel on heart rhythm, we will need a multitude of models across various levels of structural complexity (e.g., protein-affinity tests, patch clamp and single-cell electrophysiology studies, isolated heart- and animal-based research, patient testing) and even at the same level of structural complexity (e.g., test dose–response curves in cells from different parts of a heart, including pacemaker, conduction, and working myocardium, or in different species).

Thus, simplification is a central feature of model systems and determines both their utility and their limitations. Imagine, for a moment, a situation where a model captured absolutely *all* features of reality: such a "clone" would be no easier to understand than the original itself; it would lose the power to help in revealing novel insight over and beyond what is apparent from the original already and would be fraught (in biomedical research

doi: 10.1111/j.1749-6632.2011.06327.x

Ann. N.Y. Acad. Sci. 1245 (2011) 40–43 © 2011 New York Academy of Sciences.

at least) with the methodological and ethical restrictions that will have raised the need of having a model system in the first place. Those concerns are among the reasons for which we do not conduct pharmacological testing on humans before other simplified systems will have provided (simplified) answers to the likelihood of having therapeutic effects in the absence of overriding negative consequences (for a more detailed illustration, see Mirams and Noble[17]). Of course, even testing in human volunteers will not give a definitive answer on possible (in particular rare) side effects, as one human is also just a partial representation (a model) of the entire species.

From understanding models as tools that are of use for some but not all purposes (no tool ever is), the challenge arises to pick "the right one" for a purpose. This needs to be driven by an appreciation of the relevance of models in a given setting (applicability to the question at hand), their quality (e.g., in terms of representing essential features of the original, and hence supporting reproducibility of findings), and cost (not just in terms of money, but also with regard to training needs and ethical considerations). Everything else being equal, *models should be as simple as possible, yet as complex as necessary to address a given question.*[4]

While all of the above applies equally to conceptual, experimental, and computational models, the development and validation of the latter is an area that deserves further discussion. It is easy to regard bio-mathematical modeling as any of a wide range of activities: (i) completely futile because of the complexity of biological systems; (ii) an exercise in restating what we already know; (iii) a necessary and complementary component to other research tools; and presumably many more.

It is easy to sympathize with (i), given that there is so much we do not yet know about biological structures and functions and their dynamic interplay. Even the data we already have obtained are often not included in model representations, in part because of genuine arguments in favor of simplification and in part because we do not have the algorithms and computing power to extract and use relevant information. In that sense, statement (ii) is only half-true, at best. It is also at least half-wrong, as the complexity of multiple feed-forward and feed-back pathways in complex biological systems (see (i)) can be hard to penetrate or know, even if we have the relevant underlying information. Computer models, with their

capability of observing basic laws, such as conservation of mass, charge, and momentum, are a potentially amazing aide in the knowledge-generation process. Of course, all a computer model can do (at best) is to offer an assessment of *plausibility*. This argues in favor of (iii), as different types of models should be used in direct iteration, with experimental data providing input for both model generation and validation.

One goal of systems biology, therefore, would appear to be the generation of models that are relevant for the range of questions we need to address, representative of the reality we wish to capture, reproducible and robust, and reasonable in terms of the different facets of costs involved.[3] A good illustration of how this view is starting to change the way we conduct biomedical investigations is the European Community-funded Virtual Physiological Human (VPH) initiative, which is focused on developing and implementing biophysically based computational models to aid clinically relevant research and development.[5] The success of this initiative, which forms part of the worldwide Physiome effort (http://www.physiome.org.nz/), has been based on the integration of vast arrays of data, to extract information, and to turn this into practically applicable knowledge related to various parts and processes of the human body. One of the most prominent examples of the successful use of this approach has been the modeling of the heart.

Cardiac computational modeling has benefited from the fact that it targets an organ whose function displays a high degree of spatial and temporal regularity, for which a wealth of high-quality structural and functional data exists at multiple levels of spatio-temporal integration (including, for example, histology, computed tomography, magnetic resonance imaging, patch clamp, and electrocardiology). Its leading position among organ models is also related to the long history of computational modeling (from the first biophysically based cell models in the 1960s, to bulk three-dimensional (3D) geometry models in the 1990s, and most recently, highly detailed histo-anatomical models) and to the high relevance of this as a target for biomedical exploration. This has led to highly successful uses of computational modeling as a predictive tool, for instance in the assessment of pharmacological effects on the heart. Thus, Mirams *et al.* performed simulations using cellular models that integrated preclinical information on multi-channel block for various pharmacological compounds, showing that this could be used to improve the reliability of early cardiac safety prediction beyond current methods.[6] In another recent example, Moreno *et al.* used similar models to simulate the interaction kinetics of the anti-arrhythmic drugs flecainide and lidocaine with cardiac sodium channels, predicting clinically relevant concentrations at which flecainide and lidocaine will exacerbate, rather than ameliorate, arrhythmia.[7] These studies illustrate effective virtual drug-screening, using models of drug–channel interactions, to predict the effects of pharmacological compounds on heart rhythm and, hence, clinical utility and marketability.

Even though the above examples illustrate that heart models are becoming predictive, much remains to be done in this field. Thus, while modern histo-anatomically structured "heart" models are now based on imaging data at *para*-cellular resolution,[8] they do not usually include the atria or the big vessels, most of them are static (i.e., not considering the all-essential pump function of the heart), and very few represent any cell population other than myocytes (even though cardiac nonmyocytes, mainly fibroblasts, outnumber muscle cells even in the healthy heart, with potentially important functions beyond structural support roles usually ascribed to connective tissue[9]).

Going down in structural complexity, the above advances in 3D models that incorporate structural detail in the micro-to-macro domain (cell to organ) are not yet matched by representations in the nano-to-micro range (protein / membrane systems to whole cell). Arguably, the lack of insight into 3D nano-structures is one of the current bottlenecks on the way to bridging insight from subcellular networks to systems' behavior. This is being addressed now using advanced nanoscopic imaging modalities, such as electron microscopic tomography (based on back-projecting multiple 2D electron microscopy images, obtained over a wide range of viewing directions, to reproduce 3D data sets with a resolution of ∼5 nm or better, sufficient to visualize macromolecular assemblies)[10] and interferometric photoactivated localization microscopy (combination of photoactivated localization microscopy with single-photon, simultaneous multiphase interferometry that provides sub-20 nm 3D protein local-

ization with high molecular specificity).[11] It stands to expect, therefore, that we will have highly structured 3D models of cells to support spatially resolved simulation of intracellular activity before the end of this decade.

Combined, this poses an enormous challenge, requiring dynamic structure–function data that span huge spatial and temporal domains (on the order of 10^{-9}–10^0 m from ion channel pore to whole body, and 10^{-9}–10^7 s from protein configuration changes to disease development). In addition, there is a need for a unified set (or, at least, for a set of definitions to allow interaction)[12] of nondeterministic computational models accounting for variability and stochastic behavior at multiple levels of structural and functional complexity. An essential, but currently lacking, instrument for seamless incorporation of cardiac experimental data into computational models is a clearly defined minimum information standard to govern recording, annotating, and reporting of data. Attempts to establish reporting standards that are acceptable to (and, hence, hopefully adhered to by) the greater research community are currently occurring across many scientific disciplines. For cardiac electrophysiological experimentation specifically, a standard for reporting Minimum Information for a Cardiac Electrophysiology Experiment (MICEE) was proposed in the autumn of 2011.[13] The ultimate goal of MICEE is to develop a useful interface that facilitates dissemination of the minimum information necessary for reproduction of cardiac electrophysiology research, allowing for easier comparison and utilization of findings by others (including computational modelers). Improving experimental and theoretical modelling techniques across the above spatio-temporal ranges, and implementing reporting and dissemination standards, could be perceived as "mission impossible." We would argue that it is "mission imperative," as there is simply no alternative to the quantitative study of dynamic structure–function interactions in complex systems if we wish to advance, and make more efficient, biomedical research and development.

As mentioned above, state-of-the-art computational modeling needs continuous iteration with experimental (both basic and clinical) research to avoid tapping into the *plausibility trap*, by which a quantitatively plausible explanation is taken for proof of a matter. Computational models are useful for hypothesis formation, for guiding experimental approaches, and for data analysis and interpretation, but the proof of the pudding is in the eating. In fact, when computational models *fail* to reproduce observed behavior, they can be most useful for the stimulation of new insight, as it is when our best-conceived expectations are proven wrong that we learn the most. Such "failures" in theoretical models can drive novel biomedical research, to determine whether input data, boundary conditions, interpretations, or model implementations are missing relevant aspects. As an illustration of this iterative approach, the studies by Lei and Kohl[14] and Cooper *et al.*[15] into stretch-induced acceleration of cardiac pacemaker function initially explored the effects of cell swelling (considered, at the time, as a suitable experimental model of stretch), finding an unexpected slowing of pacemaker rate. This was explained using computational models and highlighted the limitations of the original experimental technique. A new experimental approach to axially stretch pacemaker cells was then applied, which indeed revealed the expected rate acceleration, known to occur in native tissue. The compatibility of cell electrophysiological responses with tissue behavior was explored in further computational modeling, and a stretch-activated ion channel was identified as a plausible substrate underlying the response. This example demonstrates how computational and experimental models, if conducted in direct iteration, can advance our understanding of biological systems. It also highlights the role that advanced engineering techniques play in this setting (they are for *reduction* what computational modeling is for *integration*).

To conclude, systems biology is a valuable approach to biomedical research, with the potential to identify the dynamic cross-talk between *entity* and *parts*, as they affect each other through structural and functional interaction across all levels relevant for biomedicine. This is the hype. Models, used in this discovery process, are simplified representations of reality. This is reflected in the popular quote by George Box, "All models are wrong."[16] What is usually forgotten is his additional comment: ". . . the practical question is how wrong do they have to be to not be useful."[16] The art, therefore, lies in the appropriate matching of tasks and tools, and systems biology is helping us in getting better at doing that. This is the hope.

Conflicts of interest

The authors declare no conflicts of interest.

References

1. Kohl, P., E.J. Crampin, T.A. Quinn & D. Noble. 2010. Systems biology: an approach. *Clin. Pharmacol. Ther.* **88:** 25–33.
2. von Bertalanffy, L. 1968. *General System Theory.* George Braziller, Inc. New York.
3. Kohl, P. & D. Noble. 2009. Systems biology and the virtual physiological human. *Mol. Syst. Biol.* **5:** 292.
4. Garny, A., D. Noble & P. Kohl. 2005. Dimensionality in cardiac modelling. *Prog. Biophys. Mol. Biol.* **87:** 47–66.
5. Hunter, P., P.V. Coveney, B. de Bono, V. Diaz, *et al.* 2010. A vision and strategy for the VPH in 2010 and beyond. *Phil. Trans. Roy. Soc. A.* **368:** 2595–2614.
6. Mirams, G.R., Y. Cui, A. Sher, M. Fink, *et al.* 2011. Simulation of multiple ion channel block provides improved early prediction of compounds' clinical torsadogenic risk. *Cardiovasc. Res.* **91:** 53–61.
7. Moreno, J.D., Z.I. Zhu, P.C. Yang & J.R. Bankston. 2011. A computational model to predict the effects of class I antiarrhythmic drugs on ventricular rhythms. *Sci. Transl. Med.* **31:** 98ra83.
8. Plank, G., R.A.B. Burton, P. Hales, M. Bishop, *et al.* 2009. Generation of histo-anatomically representative models of the individual heart: tools and application. *Philos. Transact. A. Math. Phys. Eng. Sci.* **367:** 2257–2292.
9. Camelliti, P., T. Borg & P. Kohl. 2005. Structural and functional characterisation of cardiac fibroblasts. *Cardiovasc. Res.* **65:** 40–51.
10. Iribe, G., C.W. Ward, P. Camelliti, C. Bollensdorff, *et al.* 2009. Axial stretch of rat single ventricular cardiomyocytes causes an acute and transient increase in Ca^{2+} spark rate. *Circ. Res.* **104:** 787–795.
11. Shtengel, G., J.A. Galbraith, C.G. Galbraith, J. Lippincott-Schwartz, *et al.* 2009. Interferometric fluorescence superresolution microscopy resolves 3D cellular ultrastructure. *Proc. Natl. Acad. Sci. USA* **106:** 3125–3130.
12. Kohl, P., P.J. Hunter & R.L. Winslow. 2011. Model interactions: 'It is the simple, which is so difficult.' *Prog. Biophys. Mol. Biol.* **107:** 1–3.
13. Quinn, T.A., S. Granite, M.A. Allessie, C. Antzelevitch, *et al.* 2011. Minimum Information about a Cardiac Electrophysiology Experiment (MICEE): standardised reporting for model reproducibility, interoperability, and data sharing. *Prog. Biophys. Mol. Biol.* **107:** 4–10.
14. Lei, M. & P. Kohl. 1998. Swelling-induced decrease in spontaneous pacemaker activity of rabbit isolated sino-atrial node cells. *Acta. Physiol. Scand.* **164:** 1–12.
15. Cooper, P.J., M. Lei, L.X. Cheng & P. Kohl. 2000. Axial stretch increases spontaneous pacemaker activity in rabbit isolated sino-atrial node cells. *J. Appl. Physiol.* **89:** 2099–2104.
16. Box, G.E.P. & N.R. Draper. 1986. *Empirical Model-Building and Response Surfaces.* John Wiley & Sons, Inc. New York.
17. Mirams, G.R. & D. Noble. 2011. Is it time for *in silico* simulation of drug cardiac side effects? *Ann. N.Y. Acad. Sci.* **1245:** 44–47.

Ann. N.Y. Acad. Sci. ISSN 0077-8923

ANNALS OF THE NEW YORK ACADEMY OF SCIENCES
Issue: *Animal Models: Their Value in Predicting Drug Efficacy and Toxicity*

Is it time for *in silico* simulation of drug cardiac side effects?

Gary R. Mirams[1] and Denis Noble[2]

[1]Department of Computer Science, University of Oxford, Oxford, United Kingdom. [2]Department of Physiology, Anatomy & Genetics, University of Oxford, United Kingdom

Address for correspondence: Gary Mirams, Department of Computer Science, University of Oxford, Parks Road, Oxford, OX1 3QD, UK. gary.mirams@cs.ox.ac.uk

Cardiac simulation is used to integrate information on drug action to predict side effects on the whole heart. Could simulation begin to replace animal models?

Keywords: torsade de pointes; cardiac toxicity; computer modeling; hERG

For many years, a large focus of cardiac safety pharmacology has been on the prediction of whether a compound is likely to induce a particular type of cardiac ventricular arrhythmia, called torsade de pointes (TdP). TdP is often exceedingly rare, occurring perhaps only once in 10,000 patient years of therapeutic use; however, it can be fatal, as the TdP arrhythmia can degenerate into ventricular fibrillation and cause sudden cardiac death. The rarity means that it is extremely difficult to screen for this liability during clinical trials, and this potential severity has led to TdP becoming a leading cause of drug withdrawal from the market.

Since TdP is observed so rarely in practice, we rely on other biomarkers that have been associated with an increased TdP risk, which are more easily observed.[1] One of these is blockade of the human Ether-a-go-go Related Gene (hERG) channel, which is responsible for carrying the rapidly activating potassium current (I_{Kr}).[2] I_{Kr} block causes a reduction in the repolarizing current and prolongation of the cellular action potential. At the organ or whole-body level, this is manifest as a prolongation of the QT interval of the electrocardiogram. QT prolongation is also associated with (but is neither necessary nor sufficient for) both increased TdP risk and increased risk of sudden cardiac death.[3] It is worth noting that TdP can only be diagnosed when the patient is monitored by an electrocardiogram, and so some cases of sudden cardiac death occurring outside a hospital environment may have been preceded by TdP events. Pharmaceutical companies now employ a wide range of *in vitro* and *in vivo* animal models to detect hERG block and QT prolongation at different stages of compound development. These may include, but are not limited to, isolated rabbit/guinea-pig/rat/dog myocytes, rabbit/dog Purkinje fiber, rabbit/dog ventricular wedge, Langendorff heart preparations, and *in vivo* rat/rabbit/dog/primate studies.

Redfern *et al.* correlated the degree of hERG blockade that drugs cause with the human clinical TdP risk they induce.[4] They concluded that a safety factor of a 30-fold difference between the effective therapeutic plasma concentration and the concentration of the drug that blocks hERG by 50% is advisable. However, there were a number of drugs that have been on the market for many years that were exceptions to this rule. For example, verapamil is a strong hERG blocker at therapeutic concentrations, but it has not been associated with an increased TdP risk.

Drug block of multiple ion channels may explain some of the discrepancies that appear when considering only hERG block. In oversimplified terms, block of a depolarizing current at a similar level to block of a repolarizing current may have little overall effect on the cellular action potential. Hence, a drug compound may have little effect at the tissue/whole-organ scale,

doi: 10.1111/j.1749-6632.2011.06324.x

Ann. N.Y. Acad. Sci. 1245 (2011) 44–47 © 2011 New York Academy of Sciences.

despite a strong effect on individual currents. To quantify this concept, we have turned to biophysically based mathematical models of cardiac electrophysiology. These models predict the formulation of the cellular action potential (transmembrane voltage through time) from individual ionic currents (which are themselves voltage and time dependent). These models now represent over 50 years of iteration between experiment and theory, and they encapsulate the sum of our understanding of the electrical basis for the heart's activity.[5] Such a multiple ion-channel effect was observed with ranolazine, a novel antiangina compound, which exhibits block of both hERG and the late/persistent sodium current. Computational modelling work was able to provide a mechanism by which ranolazine's strong multiple channel block led to a smaller action potential prolongation than might have been expected when considering only hERG, together with a reduction in the proarrhythmic properties that such a prolongation usually confers.[6]

Pharmaceutical companies have realized the importance of multiple ion-channel effects and typically now screen a panel of ion channel targets. In a recent study, we used data generated on three ion channels by GlaxoSmithKline (hERG, fast sodium, and L-type calcium), together with recent biophysical computer models of ventricular myocytes, to simulate the effect of multiple ion-channel block for a significant number of compounds.[7] The results suggest that prolongation of the resulting simulated action potential is linked to increased TdP risk. The method correctly classified the TdP risk of strong multiple channel blockers, such as verapamil, which have been misclassified by previous hERG-only based metrics.

Animal models are still invaluable in drug safety testing when one or more (usually both) of the following apply:

(i)   there are a number of unknown drug actions— the drug binds to a number of targets, which we cannot hope to screen without a representation of all of the possible targets in the whole system (with an animal model); or

(ii) the system we are interested in is "too complicated" to predict a drug effect—even given the list of drug targets and affinities, the whole physiological system of nonlinear reactions and feedback must be well represented (again, with an animal model).

The advent of high-throughput expression-system cell line screens offers the possibility of detecting all common cardiac ion-channel drug targets routinely, and relatively cheaply. This addresses the first point, that we can now gather enough quantitative information about compound [off-]targets to capture the significant interactions. Mathematical models, quantifying the complex interplay and feedback involved in ionic currents and generation of membrane voltage, offer the possibility of addressing the second point. There is, therefore, no major obstacle to the use of mathematical models in routine screening for cardiac side effects, and there are many benefits.

First, simulations can be run as soon as ion-channel data become available, which is usually at an early stage with larger numbers of candidate compounds than it is economical to screen with animal models. Second, these simulations are very cheap to run in terms of time, money, and resources— modern desktop computers can easily simulate a cellular action potential for thousands of paces within a minute. Third, the process can be completely automated (for a simple model of drug action), and results can be stored alongside experimental results in pharmaceutical databases. Academics are currently working with pharmaceutical partners to provide such implementations as a proof of concept to begin evaluating their predictive power. Fourth, and possibly most importantly, by offering a simplification of the complete animal/system, the mathematical models offer the hope of unpicking the precise mechanisms at play so that the whole system is not just well represented, but well understood. By understanding the mechanisms underlying TdP initiation, we may be in a position to propose safety tests for TdP that are more accurate than simply QT prolongation.[6]

We do not expect that the first attempts at this simulation of cardiac risk will be perfectly accurate; there will always be novel targets and drug interactions to consider, and the mathematical models are simplifications of reality. Thus, simulation will not completely replace animal-based cardiac safety testing. But it is worth noting that many of the existing animal model screens provide accurate predictions for human QT prolongation for only around 70% of compounds. Simulation does not, therefore, need to be 99% accurate to be useful; a method, which was predictive for 75% of compounds, could potentially replace one of the animal screens mentioned earlier, saving time, money, and resources and providing more accurate predictions earlier in drug development.

But there is also a strong case to be made for simulation and experiment to be performed in tandem, with simulation refining the information gained from the experiment. Agreement between simulation and experimental results would suggest that the majority of important drug interactions with ion channels have been captured, and that the mechanisms of the drug's action are understood. Where there is disagreement between simulation and experiment the simulation studies may be able to suggest other possible explanations for the observed behavior—for example, drug interaction with a channel that is not screened.

At the conclusion of a recent European Commission funded project on the prediction of drug impact in cardiac toxicity, a workshop was held with computational modelers, members of pharmaceutical companies, and regulatory agencies, including the U.S. Food and Drug Administration and the European Medicines Agency. A number of challenges and possibilities were raised,[8] some of which we highlight here.

Access to drug data can be a problem, with many datasets residing inside pharmaceutical companies; new initiatives such as the ILSI-HESI consortium (http://www.hesiglobal.org) are invaluable in this regard. One concern is that safety pharmacology data available in the public domain are typically summary statistics, and additional parameters and information can often be gleaned from detailed raw data. For many new drugs, with multiple ion-channel data and thorough QT study results available, postmarketing experience is presently insufficient to comment on their proarrhythmic risk. Conversely, older drugs with a well-established risk usually lack multiple ion-channel data and a thorough QT study. There are also challenges in computational modeling, with regard to consistency between different models, open-access simulation software, and publishing of models and protocols to ensure accuracy and reproducibility.[9,10]

Once these challenges have been overcome, a number of possibilities exist. During early-stage investigations, it should be possible to predict safety concerns and results of later safety tests—as discussed above with regard to refining, reducing, and replacing animal experiments. The industry could return to drugs that have been discarded because of hERG affinity but which may have a combined ion-channel action that is not cardiotoxic. Detailed studies, such as the one performed for ranolazine,[6] allow understanding of complex mechanisms of drug action, which may strengthen a dossier for submission to regulatory authorities. TdP is frequently linked to coadministration of multiple drug compounds. It is clearly not feasible to perform a human trial for every possible coadministration combination, but such a study may be possible *in silico* and would highlight drug combinations that should be avoided. In the future, as biophysical models for patient subgroups are developed (e.g., for gender, genetic syndromes, and disease states), *in silico* models may help to stratify patients according to risk for particular drugs.

In summary, we believe that the time is right to evaluate the role that *in silico* biophysical cardiac simulation can play in cardiac drug safety testing and to trial and evaluate its use inside the pharmaceutical compound development process. In addition to predicting the results of existing safety tests, *in silico* biophysical models can also be used to gain a better understanding of drug action and should be used to both design and perform novel, and more accurate, safety tests.

Conflicts of interest

GRM has received research support from Glaxo-SmithKline Plc.

References

1. Corrias, A. *et al.* 2010. Arrhythmic risk biomarkers for the assessment of drug cardiotoxicity: from experiments to computer simulations. *Philos. Transact. A. Math. Phys. Eng. Sci.* **368:** 3001–3025.
2. Pollard, C.E. *et al.* 2010. An introduction to QT interval prolongation and non-clinical approaches to assessing and reducing risk. *Br. J. Pharmacol.* **159:** 12–21.
3. Straus, S.M.J.M. *et al.* 2005. Non-cardiac QTc-prolonging drugs and the risk of sudden cardiac death. *Eur. Heart. J.* **26:** 2007–2012.
4. Redfern, W.S. *et al.* 2003. Relationships between preclinical cardiac electrophysiology, clinical QT interval prolongation and torsade de pointes for a broad range of drugs: evidence for a provisional safety margin in drug development. *Cardiovasc. Res.* **58:** 32–45.
5. Noble, D. & Y. Rudy. 2001. Models of cardiac ventricular action potentials: iterative interaction between experiment and simulation. *Philos. Transact. A. Math. Phys. Eng. Sci.* **359:** 1127–1142.

6. Noble, D. & P.J. Noble. 2006. Late sodium current in the pathophysiology of cardiovascular disease: consequences of sodium-calcium overload. *Heart* **92:** 1–5.

7. Mirams, G.R. *et al.* 2011. Simulation of multiple ion channel block provides improved early prediction of compounds' clinical torsadogenic risk. *Cardiovas. Res.* **91:** 53–61.

8. Fletcher, K. *et al.* 2011. Novel approaches to assessing cardiac safety-proceedings of a workshop: regulators, industry and academia discuss the future of in silico cardiac modelling to predict the proarrhythmic safety of drugs. *Drug Safety* **34:** 439–443.

9. Cooper, J., G.R. Mirams & S. Niederer. 2011. High throughput functional curation of cellular models. *Prog. Biophys. Mol. Biol.* **107:** 11–20.

10. Pitt-Francis, J. *et al.* 2009. Chaste: a test-driven approach to software development for biological modelling. *Comput. Phys. Commun.* **180:** 2452–2471.

Ann. N.Y. Acad. Sci. ISSN 0077-8923

Human stem cell-derived cardiomyocytes for pharmacological and toxicological modeling

Sian E. Harding

The National Heart and Lung Institute, Imperial College, London, United Kingdom

Address for correspondence: Sian E. Harding, Professor of Cardiac Pharmacology, The National Heart and Lung Institute, Imperial College, Flowers Building, 4th Floor, Armstrong Road, London SW7 2AZ, UK. sian.harding@imperial.ac.uk

Cardiomyocytes derived from human pluripotent stem cells have advantages for modeling in terms of phenotype, longevity in culture, ease of transfection, and high-throughput capability.

Keywords: stem cell; *in vitro*; cardiomyocyte; high throughput

The search for improved, humanized *in vitro* models for disease has led to a focus on human stem cell derivatives. This has been especially true for the cardiac field, where previous lack of cell lines with a true ventricular phenotype had led to a dependence on freshly isolated primary cardiomyocytes. Postnatal myocytes in culture do not grow to confluence (except in the specialized case of mouse and rat neonatal cells) and do not divide, and therefore cannot be passaged. Dedifferentiation occurs rapidly, accompanied by loss of the structure and function of the adult cell, which limits the useful period in culture to one to two days. It is for this reason that it has been difficult to obtain a stable cardiac cell line. Some atrial tumor lines (HL-1, H9c2) have been derived, but they have not found widespread use. In addition, the manipulation of protein expression, essential to the testing of hypotheses, is hampered because adult myocytes are difficult to transfect. This is a common problem with primary cells, but the myocyte seems to be one of the more extreme examples. DNA constructs cannot be introduced into adult myocytes in meaningful amounts, and only viral transfection is successful. The necessity for construction of a viral vector for each target severely reduces the speed of progress.

Human embryonic stem cell lines (hESC), first developed in 1998, were quickly shown to produce cardiomyocytes (CM) with spontaneous contractility and electrophysiological characteristics of the main cardiac subtypes: atrial, pacemaker, and ven-

tricular myocytes.[1,2] They were superior to the adult myocyte in that they would continue to beat in culture for months and could be readily transfected using plasmid or siRNA constructs.[3] Since their discovery, efforts in laboratories, including our own, have characterized hESC-CM in detail in terms of electrophysiology, calcium handling, receptor response, growth, proliferation, and survival. More recently, very similar cells to hESC have been produced by induction of pluripotency in adult somatic cells such as fibroblasts.[4] As well as avoiding any ethical concerns, induced pluripotent stem cells (iPSC) have the advantage that patient- or subject-specific cells can be derived much more easily, opening up the potential for a wide range of genotypes to be compared. iPSC can be differentiated into cardiomyocytes using similar methods to hESC, and initial results suggest that iPSC-CM and hESC-CM have very similar characteristics.[5]

The initial focus for hESC- or iPSC-derived CM, called human pluripotent stem cell-derived CM (hPSC-CM), has been to mimic acute cardiac responses, with the aim of producing models to investigate contractile impairment or arrhythmias or for using cells as a screen to detect acute cardiotoxicity of experimental compounds. A particular success has been with the modeling of arrhythmias secondary to prolongation of action potential direction (long QT syndrome), now shown in hPSC-CM derived from a number of patients with ion channel mutations.[6] From a pharmaceutical company perspective, this

doi: 10.1111/j.1749-6632.2011.06328.x

is exciting because all compounds are screened under legislative requirements for long QT by human ether-a-go-go related gene (HERG) channel blockade. It is thought that studying ion current changes in the context of a human ventricular action potential will increase the accuracy of prediction. These assays are becoming a commercial reality, with companies such as Cellular Dynamics selling iPSC-CM (iCell™) for drug candidate toxicity screening.

The utility of hPSC-CM for modeling of longer-term cardiotoxicity, for example, cardiotoxicity produced by chemotherapeutic agents, is more difficult to predict. Much of the undetected toxicity of antitumor agents is likely to be related to their long-term proapoptotic or antiangiogenic effects and antiproliferative actions on stem cells, as outlined above, rather than acute electrophysiological phenomena. It could be argued that these immature and proliferative cells do not resemble the adult myocardium, which contains terminally differentiated cardiomyocytes, unable to proliferate but susceptible to hypertrophy and necrosis/apoptosis. However, with time (weeks to months) in culture, various aspects of the hPSC-CM come to resemble those of adult cardiomyocytes, including development of SR Ca^{+2} stores, action potential configuration, and close-down of proliferative pathways. We have shown that pathways known to mediate hypertrophy or apoptosis are similar in hPSC-CM to those in adult cardiomyocytes and are induced by similar stimuli.[7] The adult heart also contains a small population of proliferating cardiac stem cells, and very recent evidence suggests that they may be particularly susceptible to damage by chemotherapeutic agents.[8] It is not known what proportional effect of the cardiotoxicity this represents. Furthermore, in hearts with a degree of disease, often found in the target clinical population, there is regression of myocytes to an immature fetal phenotype in a number of aspects (e.g., calcium handling, resistance to hypoxia). It is known that preexisting cardiac disease increases sensitivity to chemotherapeutic cardiotoxicity. The fetal phenotype of hPSC-CM may, therefore, also model some aspects of failing heart.

Finally, a particular advantage of hPSC-CM for modeling is the potential to look at interactions between compounds, because synergistic effects often pose increased risks. Cardiotoxicity is particularly evident when combinations of agents are used; for example, one trial detected cardiac dysfunction of NYHA class III or IV in 27% of the group given an anthracycline cyclophosphamide and trastuzumab compared with 8% of the group given an anthracycline, and cyclophosphamide alone.[9] Recapitulating the various possible combinations in animal models is difficult and costly, whereas the high throughput capabilities of hPSC-CM are well suited to these studies.

Overall, there is immense anticipation that hPSC-CM could supply a phenotypically authentic, human genotype-specific, easily manipulable, high throughput model for both the cardiac researcher and the pharmaceutical industry. Caution is required regarding genetic and epigenetic changes during transdifferentiation and culture, but the hurdles for *in vitro* modeling are far more likely to be overcome than are those for *in vivo* cardiac repair.

Conflicts of interest

The author declares no conflicts of interest.

References

1. Kehat, I., D. Kenyagin-Karsenti, M. Snir, *et al*. 2001. Human embryonic stem cells can differentiate into myocytes with structural and functional properties of cardiomyocytes. *J. Clin. Invest*. **108:** 407–414.
2. Mummery, C., D. Ward, C.E. van den Brink, *et al*. 2002. Cardiomyocyte differentiation of mouse and human embryonic stem cells. *J. Anat*. **200:** 233–242.
3. Braam, S.R., C. Denning, B.S. van den, *et al*. 2008. Improved genetic manipulation of human embryonic stem cells. *Nat. Methods* **5:** 389–392.
4. Yu, J., M.A. Vodyanik, K. Smuga-Otto, *et al*. 2007. Induced pluripotent stem cell lines derived from human somatic cells. *Science* **318:** 1917–1920.
5. Zwi, L., O. Caspi, G. Arbel, *et al*. 2009. Cardiomyocyte differentiation of human induced pluripotent stem cells. *Circulation* **120:** 1513–1523.
6. Matsa, E., D. Rajamohan, E Dick, *et al*. 2011. Drug evaluation in cardiomyocytes derived from human induced pluripotent stem cells carrying a long QT syndrome type 2 mutation. *Eur. Heart. J*. **32:** 952–962.
7. Foldes, G., M. Mioulane, J.S. Wright, *et al*. 2011. Modulation of human embryonic stem cell-derived cardiomyocyte growth: a testbed for studying human cardiac hypertrophy? *J. Mol. Cell Cardiol*. **50:** 367–376.
8. De Angelis, A., E. Piegari, D. Cappetta, *et al*. 2010. Anthracycline cardiomyopathy is mediated by depletion of the cardiac stem cell pool and is rescued by restoration of progenitor cell function. *Circulation* **121:** 276–292.
9. Slamon, D.J., B. Leyland-Jones, S. Shak, *et al*. 2001. Use of chemotherapy plus a monoclonal antibody against HER2 for metastatic breast cancer that overexpresses HER2. *N. Engl. J. Med*. **344:** 783–792.

Ann. N.Y. Acad. Sci. ISSN 0077-8923

Humanized mice as a preclinical tool for infectious disease and biomedical research

Leonard D. Shultz,[1] Michael A. Brehm,[2] Sina Bavari,[3] and Dale L. Greiner[2]

[1]The Jackson Laboratory, Bar Harbor, Maine. [2]University of Massachusetts Medical School, Worcester, Massachusetts. [3]USAMRIID, Fort Detrick, Maryland

Address for correspondence: Leonard D. Shultz, The Jackson Laboratory, 600 Main Street, Bar Harbor, ME 04609. lenny.shultz@jax.org

Immunodeficient mice bearing an *IL2ry^null* mutation permit engraftment of a functional human immune system and study of human-specific infectious agents that was not previously possible.

Keywords: SCID; humanized mice; immunity; infectious disease; NSG

Introduction

There is a critical need for the development of new animal models for the *in vivo* study of human immunity. Most experimental work is done in rodent models. However, mice are not humans, and observations made in rodents may not translate to the clinic. Tractable small animal models that can be engrafted with functional human cells, tissues, and immune systems would provide important predictive preclinical models to study human immunity. Moreover, there are many infectious agents that are in need of small animal models for investigation of their *in vivo* pathogenesis and for testing new drugs or vaccines that can prevent or ameliorate disease without putting individuals at risk. Many of the infectious diseases of humans are caused by organisms that do not infect mice or other laboratory animal species, precluding the study of these pathogens in traditional animal models. To address this, immunodeficient mice have been developed that can be engrafted with functional human cells, tissues, and a functional human immune system.

History of humanized mouse development

In 1983, discovery of the severe combined immunodeficiency (*Prkdc^scid*, abbreviated *scid*) mutation in CB17 mice was followed by observations that human hematopoietic cells, including peripheral blood mononuclear cells and hematopoietic stem cells (HSCs), could engraft in these mice. However, levels of engraftment were low because of genetic limitations inherent in the strain background and high levels of natural killer (NK) cells. In 1995, NOD-*scid* mice were developed that exhibit low levels of NK cells and other innate immune defects that permitted enhanced engraftment of human hematolymphoid cells.[1]

IL2ry^null and signal regulatory protein alpha (*Sirpα*): key improvements in humanized mice

A major advancement in the field was the development of immunodeficient mice bearing a targeted mutation in the IL-2 receptor common gamma chain (*IL2ry^null*).[1] These mice support enhanced engraftment of human hematopoietic cells and for the first time a fully functional human immune system.

Another key finding was discovery of the role that signal regulatory protein alpha (Sirpα) modulates human hematopoietic cell engraftment in immunodeficient mice.[1] Macrophages in NOD mice express a *Sirpα* that closely resembles human *Sirpα* and displays reduced levels of phagocytosis of human cells relative to macrophages derived from C57BL/6 and BALB/c mice that have a *Sirpα* with little homology to human *Sirpα*. This observation is likely one of the key reasons that NOD-*scid IL2ry^null* (NSG) and NOD-*Rag1^null IL2ry^null* (NRG) mice engraft at higher levels than do

doi: 10.1111/j.1749-6632.2011.06310.x

BALB/c-*Rag2*[null] *IL2rγ*[null] (BRG) mice.[2] Recently, a human *Sirpα* transgene expressed on the BRG background has been reported to exhibit enhanced engraftment of human HSC.[3]

Although *Sirpα* is a key component of determining engraftment of human hematopoietic cells in immunodeficient mice, NSG mice also have numerous defects in cells of the innate immune system,[1] and it will be important to determine if transgenic expression of human *Sirpα* increases human hematopoietic cell engraftment in NSG mice.

Immune models of humanized mice

A number of human immune model systems have been developed: Hu-PBL-SCID, Hu-SRC-SCID, SCID-Hu, and BLT.

Hu-PBL-SCID

Hu-PBL-SCID mice are established by engraftment of human peripheral blood leukocytes (PBL). This model system is ideal for the study of mature effector T cells as this is the primary cell population that engrafts. This system has also been used as a model for the study of xenogeneic graft-versus-host disease (xeno-GVHD).[4] These data document that the engrafted human T cells retain their immune function after engraftment into the immunodeficient recipient. A limitation of this model is the lack of HLA-expression in the recipient. The human T cells are educated on the PBL-donor thymus and are HLA-restricted. The antigen-presenting cells (APCs) in the NSG recipient express the mouse major histocompatibility complex (MHC), and function poorly as APCs for human T cells. Second, the mature functional human T cells that engraft mediate xeno-GVHD confounding study of the human immune function in the recipient.

Hu-SRC-SCID

Hu-SRC-SCID mice are established by intravenous or intrafemoral injection of conditioned adults, or intravenous or intrahepatic injection of conditioned newborns with human HSC. Engraftment of adult immunodeficient *IL2rγ*[null] mice with HSC leads to development of multiple hematopoietic cell lineages but few T cells.[2] In contrast, human T cells are readily generated after engraftment of newborn NSG mice with HSC.

SCID-Hu

The SCID-Hu model is established by implantation of human fetal liver and thymus fragments under the renal capsule.[1] This system was one of the first models available for the study of human immunodeficiency virus (HIV) in a small animal model, and was used extensively to evaluate potential HIV therapeutics. A major limitation of this model is the paucity of human T cells in the peripheral tissues.[1]

BLT

The BLT model system (bone marrow, liver, and thymus) is established by implantation of fetal human liver and thymus fragments under the renal capsule of irradiated recipients and intravenous injection of fetal liver cells HSC (Fig. 1). A robust human immune system develops, including human T cells that are HLA restricted. A major advantage of this model system is that a human mucosal immune system is also generated. This model has been used to establish a system for the study of mechanisms of mucosal infection with HIV, a common pathway for transmission of this virus in humans.

Limitations of immune systems in humanized mice

Limitations include (1) lack of HLA molecules required for appropriate T cell selection in the Hu-SRC-SCID or lack of appropriate HLA APCs in the BLT model; (2) species-specificity of growth factors and other molecules; (3) low levels of humoral immune responses; (4) limited development of lymph nodes; (5) few circulating human red blood cells, neutrophils, or platelets; and (6) residual innate immunity of the host.

HLA and T cell education

We and others have developed human HLA-transgenic (Tg) mice. Using NSG-HLA-A2 Tg mice engrafted with HLA-A2 HSC, we have shown that functional human immune systems develop, and that HLA-A2 restricted human CD8[+] T cells are generated following infection with dengue[5] or Epstein–Barr virus (EBV).[6]

However, NSG mice still express murine MHC class I and class II antigens. To address this, we have developed NSG mice deficient in host MHC class I and class II.[4] Adoptive transfer of PBL into NSG mice deficient in MHC class I or class II significantly delays the development of xeno-GVHD.[4] More recently, we have used these new generation NSG MHC class II–deficient mice to establish a novel model for allo-GVHD.

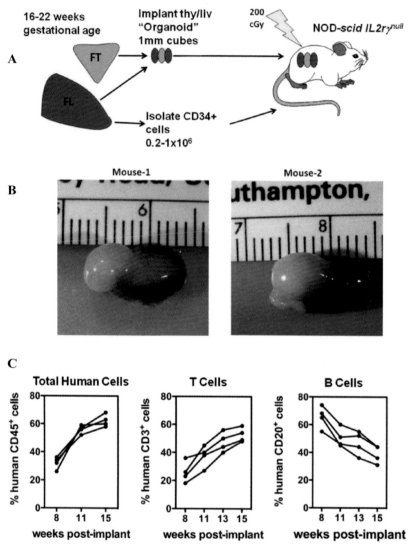

Figure 1. Establishment of the BLT model. (A) Schematic of the approach for transplantation of fragments of human fetal liver and thymus in the renal capsule followed by light irradiation of the recipient and intravenous injection of human CD34[+] HSC isolated from the same fetal liver preparation. (B and C) Thymus and T cell development in BLT mice. Representative thymus grafts 16 weeks after transplantation of (1 mm) three fragments of fetal thymus, (B). Development of human CD45[+] cells, CD3[+] T cells, and CD20[+] B cells in the blood of NSG-BLT mice, (C).

Species-specific growth factors and other molecules

A number of species-specific factors in mice are not crossreactive with human cells.[1] To address this, we and others provide recombinant proteins or use knockin and transgenic immunodeficient *IL2rγ* [null] mice expressing human cytokines, growth factors, and other human factors. For example, in the original description of NSG mice, administration of recombinant human IL-7 enhanced human T cell growth,[1] and administration of recombinant human IL-7 during the induction of a delayed hypersensitivity reaction increased the human cellular immune response in humanized mice.[7] More recently, expression of human *Sirpα* in BRG mice enhanced human cell engraftment.[3] Our laboratory has created a panel of human HLA and cytokine transgenic NSG mouse models and has additional models under development.

Human-specific infectious agents in humanized mice

HIV

HIV was the first human infectious agent to be studied in humanized mice.[1] Since the development of immunodeficient *IL2rγ* [null] mice, the use of humanized mice in infectious disease has expanded exponentially. For HIV research, the BLT model permits study of infection via the mucosal route. In these models, numerous therapeutic approaches have been used to prevent and treat infection. In the Hu-PBL-SCID and Hu-SRC-SCID models, we have used humanized NSG mice to demonstrate the therapeutic activity siRNA therapy to suppress HIV infection.[8]

Dengue virus

Humanized mice can support infection with dengue virus, and both T cell- and B cell- specific responses can be elicited.[5] Using the Hu-SRC-SCID model, we have shown the induction of anti-dengue virus antibodies, and generation of HLA-A2–restricted CD8[+] T cell responses.[5] Using Hu-SRC-SCID mice, it has also been shown that administration of siRNA against TNF-α in Hu-SRC-SCID mice infected with dengue virus suppressed the production of TNF-α by human dendritic cells. Of interest will be the study of dengue virus infection in the BLT model, which seems to generate more robust human immune responses than does the Hu-SRC-SCID or Hu-PBL-SCID model systems.

Malaria

There has been a growing need for an animal model for the study of malaria.

Early studies using *Plasmodium falciparum*–infected human erythrocyte–engrafted NOD-*scid* mice showed low levels of parasitemia. Investigators have used NSG mice to engraft human red blood cells, and induce a productive infection with *P. falciparum* for the study of efficacy of antimalarial drugs.

EBV

EBV will only infect human cells and tissues, and humanized mice have been used to study the immune response to EBV infection.[6] The use of NSG HLA-A2 Tg mice engrafted with HLA-A2 CD34[+] cells derived from umbilical cord blood permitted the identification of CD8[+] HLA-A2–restricted T cell responses to EBV epitopes.[6]

Salmonella typhi

Using the NSG Hu-SRC-SCID model, humanized mice can be infected with this pathogen, and this induced a lethal outcome with pathological and inflammatory cytokine responses resembling human typhoid.[9] This model was used to identify potential Salmonella virulence determinants that modulated their *in vivo* infectivity. Another model of *S. typhi* based on the BRG strain in the Hu-SRC-SCID model also supported productive infection, but the infection in this strain was not lethal, permitting the immune response to *S. typhi* to be investigated.

We are also developing humanized mouse models of hemorrhagic fever virus infection that is emerging as a serious biological threat. These examples of how humanized mice are being used to study human-specific infectious agents without putting individuals at risk suggest that there will be a growing interest in these models for such studies. Indeed, we have been able to substantiate the use of these models to accurately determine efficacy of antiviral agents against highly deadly viruses such as Ebola and Marburg. In these studies, we determined the level of viral clearance in human cells engrafted in NSG mice in presence of specific therapeutics (data not shown). These types of approaches encompass critical components of data packages for FDA consideration of licensing of therapeutics and vaccines against biological agents where human clinical studies may not be feasible or possible.

Regenerative medicine and cancer

There are multiple uses for humanized mice in translational biomedical research. For example, the function of cells and tissues derived from embryonic stem cells or induced pluripotent stem cells can be investigated *in vivo*. Humanized mice are used to identify human tumor stem cells. In particularly intriguing studies on human acute myelogenous leukemia (AML), NSG mice were engrafted with chemotherapy-resistant AML stem cells to identify the precise location of these stem cells in the bone marrow of the recipients. These studies were extended to validate the cell surface phenotype of the AML stem cells and to determine therapeutic targets for quiescent, chemotherapy-resistant leukemia stem cells. Finally, the humanized mice engrafted with these AML stem cells were used to develop a novel protocol for elimination of the leukemic stem cells, highlighting the potential of humanized mice to identify novel approaches for the clinical treatment of tumors and provide a practical guide for how to treat the disease.[10]

Summary

Immunodeficient *IL2rγ* ^{null} mice permit *in vivo* investigation of functional human cells and tissues. Humanized mice are rapidly becoming important investigative tools as preclinical models of human translational medicine. Study of functional human cells and tissues in a small animal model provides a cost-efficient approach that will bridge translation of results obtained using *in vitro* human cultures and *in vivo* studies in rodents to the clinic. Humanized mice permit investigation of human immune responses to infectious disease as well as providing a platform for testing human-specific reagents and drugs. The model systems that have been developed recently set the stage for an increasingly important role humanized mice will have in preclinical translational research on human cells and tissues.

Acknowledgments

This work was supported by National Institutes of Health research Grants AI46629 (DLG), AI73871 (DLG), CA34196 (LDS), DK089572 (DLG, LDS), a grant from USAMRAA; an institutional Diabetes Endocrinology Research Center (DERC) Grant (DK32520); a grant from the University of Massachusetts Center for AIDS Research, P30 AI042845 (MAB); and grants from the Juvenile Diabetes Research Foundation, International, the Helmsley Foundation, and USAMRIID. The contents of this publication are solely the responsibility of the authors and do not necessarily represent the official views of the National Institutes of Health.

Conflicts of interest

The authors declare no conflicts of interest.

References

1. Shultz, L.D., F. Ishikawa & D.L. Greiner. 2007. Humanized mice in translational biomedical research. *Nat. Rev. Immunol.* **7:** 118–130.
2. Brehm, M.A., A. Cuthbert, C. Yang, *et al.* 2010. Parameters for establishing humanized mouse models to study human immunity: analysis of human hematopoietic stem cell engraftment in three immunodeficient strains of mice bearing the IL2rgamma(null) mutation. *Clin. Immunol.* **135:** 84–98.
3. Strowig, T., A. Rongvaux, C. Rathinam, *et al.* 2011. Transgenic expression of human signal regulatory protein alpha in Rag2-/-{gamma}c-/- mice improves engraftment of human hematopoietic cells in humanized mice. *Proc. Natl. Acad. Sci. U. S. A.* **108:** 13218–13223.
4. King, M.A., L. Covassin, M.A. Brehm, *et al.* 2009. Hu-PBL-NOD-*scid IL2rg* ^{null} mouse model of xenogeneic graft-versus-host-like disease and the role of host MHC. *Clin Exp Immunol* **157:** 104–118.
5. Jaiswal, S., T. Pearson, H. Friberg, *et al.* 2009. Dengue virus infection and virus-specific HLA-A2 restricted immune responses in humanized NOD-scid IL2rgammanull mice. *PLoS ONE* **4:** e7251.
6. Shultz, L.D., Y. Saito, Y. Najima, *et al.* 2010. Generation of functional human T-cell subsets with HLA-restricted immune responses in HLA class I expressing NOD/SCID/IL2r gamma(null) humanized mice. *Proc. Natl. Acad. Sci. U. S. A.* **107:** 13022–13027.
7. Unsinger, J., J.S. McDonough, L.D. Shultz, *et al.* 2009. Sepsis-induced human lymphocyte apoptosis and cytokine production in "humanized" mice. *J. Leukoc. Biol.* **86:** 219–227.
8. Kumar, P., H.S. Ban, S.S. Kim, *et al.* 2008. T cell-specific siRNA delivery suppresses HIV-1 infection in humanized mice. *Cell* **134:** 577–586.
9. Libby, S.J., M.A. Brehm, D.L. Greiner, *et al.* 2010. Humanized nonobese diabetic-scid IL2rgammanull mice are susceptible to lethal Salmonella Typhi infection. *Proc. Natl. Acad. Sci. U. S. A.* **107:** 15589–15594.
10. Saito, Y., N. Uchida, S. Tanaka, *et al.* 2010. Induction of cell cycle entry eliminates human leukemia stem cells in a mouse model of AML. *Nat. Biotechnol.* **28:** 275–280.

Ann. N.Y. Acad. Sci. ISSN 0077-8923

Humanized mice for the study of type 1 and type 2 diabetes

Dale L. Greiner,[1] Michael A. Brehm,[1] Vishnu Hosur,[2] David M. Harlan,[1] Alvin C. Powers,[3] and Leonard D. Shultz[2]

[1]University of Massachusetts Medical School, Worcester, Massachusetts. [2]The Jackson Laboratory, Bar Harbor, Maine. [3]Vanderbilt University, Nashville, Tennessee

Address for correspondence: Dale L. Greiner, 373 Plantation Street, Biotech 2, Suite 218, Worcester, MA 01605. dale.greiner@umassmed.edu

The availability of immunodeficient mice engrafted with functional human immune systems and islets permits *in vivo* study of human diabetes without putting patients at risk.

Keywords: diabetes; humanized mice; animal models; islets

Introduction

Diabetes encompasses a group of diseases that have in common high glucose levels because of an absolute or relative deficiency in insulin production and/or insulin action. Diabetes is classified as type 1 (T1D), an absolute deficiency of insulin requiring administration of exogenous insulin, or type 2 (T2D), a relative deficiency of insulin and defects in insulin action. Diabetes in the United States afflicts 8.3% of the population, representing ∼26 million Americans at an annual cost of ∼$200 billion/year (http://www.unitedhealthgroup.com/hrm/UNH_WorkingPaper5.pdf).

Rodent models of diabetes have facilitated our understanding of the disease's cause and identified potential treatments. However, mice and humans differ significantly with regard to their immune systems and pancreatic islet cellular composition, function, and gene expression.[1] Moreover, investigating human T1D pathogenesis has been difficult because of the inaccessibility of the pancreas for study and the inability to analyze the interaction of immune cells with islets *in vivo*. Despite decades of study with rodent models of T1D, therapies that prevent or cure human T1D continue to elude us.

Our laboratories have focused on developing humanized mice to study diabetes pathogenesis and to test potential therapies. We define humanized mice as immunodeficient mice that are engrafted with functional human cells and tissues. This encompasses the transplantation of human islets as well as engraftment of human hematopoietic and immune systems. The need for humanized mice is clearly evident because current mouse models have not effectively predicted clinical trial outcomes in humans. In addition, there is an urgent need to investigate human-specific therapies on human cells and tissues *in vivo*. The availability of humanized mice enables clinically relevant *in vivo* studies of human cells, tissues, and immune systems without putting patients at risk.

Humanized SCID mice: a paradigm shift in diabetes research

We have created novel immunodeficient mouse strains that support engraftment with functional human tissues, including hematopoietic stem cells (HSC), mature lymphocytes, and islets. These unique strains are based on NOD-*scid* mice expressing a targeted mutation in the IL2 receptor common gamma chain ($IL2r\gamma^{null}$).[2] NOD-*scid* $IL2r\gamma^{null}$ (NSG) mice are severely immunodeficient and permit high engraftment of functional human cells and tissues.[2] This makes NSG mice ideal to investigate human immune system function *in vivo* and to identify a therapeutic intervention's mechanisms of action.

doi: 10.1111/j.1749-6632.2011.06318.x

How can we use humanized mouse models to study diabetes?

Humanized mice can be used to address the critical questions that are difficult or impossible to study in patients. First, whereas in patients the disease process can only be studied after T1D is well established, the humanized mouse can be developed to identify the disease's initiating factors. Second, the humanized mouse permits access to the immune cells not just from peripheral tissues, but also from the target organ (the pancreas) so that those immune effector populations can be studied. It is simply not possible and is unethical to biopsy the pancreas for the study pancreatic autoreactive cells in patients with T1D. Third, humanized mice will identify potential therapeutic targets and allow testing of novel therapeutics *in vivo*, without putting patients at risk.

Considerations for creating humanized mouse models of diabetes

Meaningful humanized mouse T1D models will require several limitations to be addressed. First, T1D is a T cell–mediated disease, so the islet-associated antigenic targets need to be identical between human and mouse, or in the case of human-specific diabetogenic autoantigens, transgenic expression of the autoantigen or other approaches must be used. Second, the immune cell donor and the islets within the recipient mice need to be matched at the major histocompatibility complex (MHC, in humans termed HLA). Third, a number of murine cytokines and factors do not signal through the corresponding human receptors. The models we have created have been designed to address these limitations.

Models of hyperglycemic humanized mice

Although immunodeficient mice have been used for over three decades for the study of human islets *in vivo*, the earlier models have several drawbacks. First, these early models of immunodeficient mice have natural killer (NK) cell activity.[2] Human islets are highly sensitive to NK cell killing. Second, these early models did not support engraftment with a functional human immune system. In contrast, NSG mice are completely NK cell deficient[2] and support engraftment with human islets, beta stem/progenitor cells, as well as functional human immune systems.

The most commonly used approach to study human islet function is to perform transplants into hyperglycemic mice and monitor blood glucose levels. Although injecting streptozotocin (STZ) will render the mice hyperglycemic, the response is quite variable, STZ can be toxic, and endogenous mouse beta cells sometimes recover, all of which conspire to complicate interpreting human islet graft function.

To address these concerns, we are developing new models of immunodeficient hyperglycemic mice. Mice bearing the *Ins2^Akita* mutation (so-called Akita mice) develop spontaneous hyperglycemia at three to six weeks of age because of insulin 2 protein misfolding, which induces endoplasmic reticulum stress and beta cell apoptosis. We have described NOD-*Rag1^null IL2rγ^null Ins2^Akita* (NRG-Akita) mice bearing the *Ins2^Akita* mutation. These mice spontaneously develop hyperglycemia, and normoglycemia can be restored by transplanting human islets.[3] NRG-Akita mice can also be engrafted with functional human immune systems that can reject human islet allografts.[3] We have also used NRG-Akita mice to investigate human beta cells' proliferative capacity *in vivo* under normoglycemic and hyperglycemic conditions.[4]

A second model is based on the (Tg[*RIP-HuDTR*]) mouse. Mouse cells do not bind diphtheria toxin (DT) with high affinity. Administration of DT to mice expressing the human DT receptor (DTR) under the control of the rat insulin promoter (RIP) will specifically kill the mouse beta cells and induce hyperglycemia. We have backcrossed the DTR transgene onto NSG mice. The initial characterization of NSG Tg(*RIP-HuDTR*) mice is underway. An advantage is that the hyperglycemia can be induced at will, is not associated with STZ toxicity, and is irreversible.

In some experimental designs, it may be advantageous to induce hyperglycemia and, when desired, permit the mouse beta cell function to recover. For this, we are developing the NSG Tg(*Ins-rtTA*) Tg(*TET-DTA*) strain. These mice express DT A chain (DTA) in beta cells when the *TET-DTA* gene is activated by adding doxycycline ("doxy") to the animals' drinking water.[5] Because expression of a single DTA molecule will kill the beta cell, and as most but not all of the beta cells are activated to express DTA when doxy is administered, so long as doxy is given, the mice remain hyperglycemic. And yet stopping the doxy permits the remaining beta cells to proliferate and restore normoglycemia.[5] We are currently generating these mice by speed congenic backcrossing the *Ins-rtTA and TET-DTA* transgenes onto the NSG strain.

Although it is not currently possible, practical approaches to permit islet imaging is of considerable interest for the diagnosis and prognosis of prediabetes, to determine a therapeutic intervention's efficacy, and to follow transplanted islets' fate. Humanized mice can be used to test approaches for noninvasive *in vivo* imaging of human islets. For example, we have used a novel "pretargeting" approach to image human islets engrafted in NSG mice.[6]

Immune engraftment models of NSG mice

NSG models that can be used to study human immune cell function include the Hu-PBL-SCID, Hu-SRC-SCID, and BLT (fetal hematopoietic stem cell, liver, and thymus) models.[2]

Hu-PBL-SCID mice are used to examine alloimmunity, autoimmunity, and viralimmunity.[2] However, mature human T cells retain xeno-reactivity, and upon engraftment, generate a potent graft-versus-host disease (GVHD).[7] Newer genetic modifications of NSG mice deficient in MHC class I and/or class II reduce GVHD, permitting investigation of immunity by minimizing the confounding effects of xeno-GVHD.[7]

Hu-SRC-SCID mice are established by engrafting newborn or adult NSG mice with human HSC. The advantage of this model is that essentially all of the cells of both adaptive and innate immune system engraft, and the engrafted immune system is naive. The disadvantage is that the human T cells develop in the mouse thymus and are therefore educated on mouse, not human, MHC.

BLT mice have fragments of human fetal liver and thymus engrafted under the renal capsule and are then given an intravenous injection of fetal liver HSC derived from the same donor.[2] BLT mice develop functional innate and adaptive immune systems, including all hematopoietic lineage cells. Moreover, as HSC are educated on self-MHC, they are HLA-restricted. Both the Hu-SRC-SCID and BLT model systems have been used to study many aspects of human immunobiology.[2]

We have shown that NRG-Akita mice engrafted with either PBL or with HSC will develop a functional human immune system that can reject human

islet allografts.[3,8] The next step is to engraft functional human autoimmune systems into NSG mice for the study of human autoimmunity.

New HLA genetic models of NSG mice

We have developed several Tg strains on the NSG strain background, including HLA class I and class II alleles representing up to 80% of the HLA-locus genes associated with T1D. We have also shown that NSG HLA-A2 transgenic mice engrafted with umbilical cord blood HLA-A2[+] HSC can support the development of HLA-A2–restricted CD8[+] T cells following infection with dengue[9] or Epstein–Barr virus.[10] We have also developed NSG mice deficient in mouse MHC class I and class II that eliminate education of human T cells on mouse MHC.[7]

We currently are engrafting NSG-HLA Tg mice with spleen cells obtained from T1D donors through the JDRF nPOD program (http://www.jdrfnpod.org/). We have also engrafted human CD8[+] T cell derived from a HLA-A2 T1D donor that had undergone an islet transplant. The CD8[+] T cell clone is directed against the islet-specific glucose-6-phosphatase catalytic subunit–related protein peptide that has an identical sequence in mice and humans.

To address the lack of species crossreactivity between mouse and human cytokines needed for optimal human immune function, we are generating human cytokine transgenic NSG mice. The initial human Tg mice being generated express human BAFF/BLyS, a B cell survival and differentiation factor. We have shown that administration of recombinant human BLyS to Hu-PBL-SCID mice increases human B cell survival and immunization-induced antibody production. Additional human cytokine transgenic mice are being made using bacterial artificial constructs so that appropriate human regulatory elements for the genes are provided in the mouse.

Finally, so that we might optimally generate new transgenic, knockout, and knockin NSG mice, we have available embryonic stem cells (ESC) from NOD, NSG, and NRG mice (http://research.jax.org/collaboration/escell.html). These ESC can generate chimeras, and we are currently using them to create a knockout on the NOD background.

One of the approaches being taken to study T1D in humanized mice is to combine the novel induced pluripotent stem (iPS) cell technology with the new models of humanized mice. Our goal is to use iPS cells derived from T1D donors to generate the critical cells and tissues to recapitulate a donor's T1D following engraftment into humanized mice. This would permit detailed analyses of the disease as it develops and would be a platform to not only identify the causes of T1D, but also permit therapeutic manipulation of the developing human immune system to prevent or cure T1D.

In summary, the humanized mouse model is a powerful platform to study diabetes pathogenesis and to develop better treatments. Genetic manipulation of the NSG strain has generated mice that become spontaneously hyperglycemic because of a genetic mutation or that can be readily and reversibly induced to become hyperglycemic. Into these mice, we can transplant human tissues to evaluate human islets or beta stem/progenitor cells *in vivo*. Moreover, without putting patients at risk, these mice can be engrafted with functional human immune systems, permitting the *in vivo* analysis of human beta cells during alloimmune and/or autoimmune attack. These mouse models will be valuable for investigation of diabetes pathogenesis, identification of potential therapeutic targets, and for *in vivo* evaluation of drugs before entering clinical trials.

Acknowledgments

This work was supported by grants from the VA Research Service; the National Institutes of Health research Grants AI46629, DK72473, DK66636, and DK68854; the Beta Cell Biology Consortium (DK72473, DK89572); the Vanderbilt Mouse Metabolic Phenotyping Center (DK59637); the Vanderbilt Diabetes Research and Training Center (DK20593); the University of Massachusetts Institutional Diabetes Endocrinology Research Center (DERC) grant DK32520; and grants from the Juvenile Diabetes Research Foundation International and the Helmsley Foundation. Human islets were provided by NIH- and JDRF-supported islet isolation centers and the Integrated Islet Distribution Network (http://iidp.coh.org/). Human spleen samples were provided by the JDRF Network for Pancreatic Organ Donors with Diabetes (nPOD). The contents of this publication are solely the responsibility of the authors and do not necessarily represent the official views of the National Institutes of Health.

Conflicts of interest

The authors declare no conflicts of interest.

References

1. Brissova, M., M.J. Fowler, W.E. Nicholson, *et al.* 2005. Assessment of human pancreatic islet architecture and composition by laser scanning confocal microscopy. *J. Histochem. Cytochem.* **53:** 1087–1097.
2. Shultz, L.D., F. Ishikawa & D.L. Greiner. 2007. Humanized mice in translational biomedical research. *Nat. Rev. Immunol.* **7:** 118–130.
3. Brehm, M.A., R. Bortell, P. DiIorio, *et al.* 2010. Human immune system development and rejection of human islet allografts in spontaneously diabetic NOD-*Rag1^{null} IL2rg^{null} Ins2^{Akita}* mice. *Diabetes* **59:** 2265–2270.
4. DiIorio, P., A. Jurczyk, C. Yang, *et al.* 2011. Hyperglycemia-induced proliferation of adult human beta cells engrafted into spontaneously diabetic immunodeficient NOD-*Rrag1^{null} IL2rg^{null} Ins2^{Akita}* mice. *Pancreas.* **40:** 1147–1149.
5. Nir, T., D.A. Melton & Y. Dor. 2007. Recovery from diabetes in mice by beta cell regeneration. *J. Clin. Invest.* **117:** 2553–2561.
6. Liu, G., S. Dou & D. Cheng, *et al.* 2011. Human islet cell MORF/cMORF pretargeting in a xenogeneic murine transplant model. *Mol. Pharm.* **8:** 767–773.
7. King, M.A., L. Covassin, M.A. Brehm, *et al.* 2009. Hu-PBL-NOD-*scid IL2rg^{null}* mouse model of xenogeneic graft-versus-host-like disease and the role of host MHC. *Clin. Exp. Immunol.* **157:** 104–118.
8. King, M., T. Pearson, L.D. Shultz, *et al.* 2008. A new Hu-PBL model for the study of human islet alloreactivity based on NOD-scid mice bearing a targeted mutation in the IL-2 receptor gamma chain gene. *Clin. Immunol.* **126:** 303–314.
9. Jaiswal, S., T. Pearson, H. Friberg, *et al.* 2009. Dengue virus infection and virus-specific HLA-A2 restricted immune responses in humanized NOD-scid IL2rgammanull mice. *PLoS ONE* **4:** e7251.
10. Shultz, L.D., Y. Saito, Y. Najima, *et al.* 2010. Generation of functional human T-cell subsets with HLA-restricted immune responses in HLA class I expressing NOD/SCID/IL2r gamma(null) humanized mice. *Proc. Natl. Acad. Sci. U. S. A.* **107:** 13022–13027.

Ann. N.Y. Acad. Sci. ISSN 0077-8923

ANNALS OF THE NEW YORK ACADEMY OF SCIENCES

Issue: *Animal Models: Their Value in Predicting Drug Efficacy and Toxicity*

Deconstructing hepatitis C virus infection in humanized mice

Marcus Dorner and Alexander Ploss

Center for the Study of Hepatitis C, Laboratory for Virology and Infectious Disease, The Rockefeller University, New York, New York

Address for correspondence: Alexander Ploss, Center for the Study of Hepatitis C, Laboratory for Virology and Infectious Disease, The Rockefeller University, 1230 York Ave, New York, NY 10065. aploss@rockefeller.edu

Hepatitis C virus is a major medical problem. Novel small-animal models are likely to accelerate the development of more effective therapeutics and a vaccine.

Keywords: hepatitis C virus; animal models; tissue engineering

Hepatitis C virus (HCV) is a positive-sense single-stranded RNA virus of the family Flaviviridae. Infection frequently becomes chronic, resulting in an estimated global burden of 130 million carriers. Chronic hepatitis C is a risk factor for severe liver disease, including fibrosis, cirrhosis, and end-stage liver failure. Disease progression can be accelerated by certain comorbidities or environmental factors, such as HIV coinfection, obesity, and frequent alcohol consumption. In the United States, HCV is one of the major etiologies for hepatocellular carcinoma and a common indicator for liver transplantation. Recently, the first direct-acting antivirals have been approved for use alongside the existing standard of care, pegylated interferon α, and ribavirin. However, HCV treatment remains associated with adverse side effects and variable success rates. Furthermore, prophylactic or therapeutic vaccines for HCV do not exist.

Understanding the HCV life cycle and the rational design of effective therapies were delayed for years by challenges in studying the virus in cell culture and animal models. HCV exhibits a very narrow host tropism, robustly infecting only humans and chimpanzees. Chimpanzees are susceptible to patient-derived virus and infectious clones and recapitulate well the natural course of infection. The ability to experimentally infect these animals has shed light on the host immune response and aided the preclinical assessment of drug and vaccine candidates. However, studies in chimpanzees are hampered by

limited availability, high costs, and ethical concerns, which have led to a ban on the use of these animals for biomedical research in most countries. As an alternative model, the tree shrew (*Tupaia*) may sustain low-level HCV infection following experimental inoculation. But viremia in this small, primate-like species is intermittent and required that the animals be immunocompromised.

To address the medical need for more effective therapeutic interventions, as well as to answer questions of basic virology, HCV pathogenesis, and correlates of protective immunity, more tractable *in vivo* platforms are needed. Several different approaches are currently being pursued. Efforts focus on the adaptation of the virus to infect previously nonpermissive species and on engineering the cellular environment to become more permissive. Because of the ease of genetic manipulations, host adaptation approaches have primarily focused on rodents. Humanization of the host can be achieved by introducing relevant human tissue compartments—that is, the liver and a human hematopoietic system—or by genetically overcoming barriers limiting the HCV life cycle in mice (Fig. 1).

Adaptation of HCV to nonhuman hosts

HCV uses multiple cellular entry factors, including glycosaminoglycans; the low-density lipoprotein receptor; the high-density lipoprotein receptor scavenger receptor class B type I (SCARB1);

doi: 10.1111/j.1749-6632.2011.06317.x

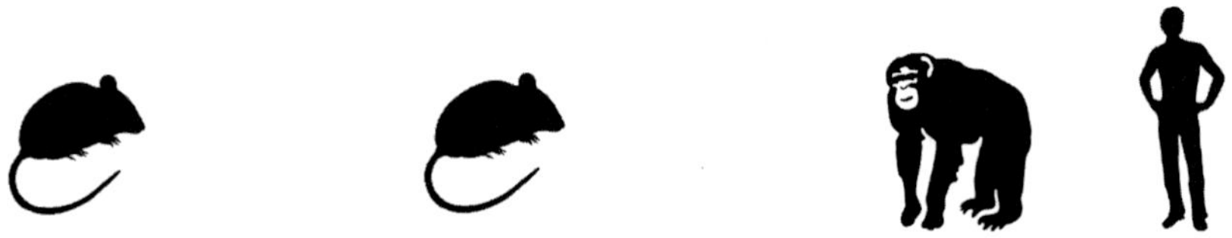

Figure 1. A multipronged approach toward animal models for HCV infection.

Approach	Mice Viral adaptation	Humanized mice genetic humanization	xenotransplantation	Chimpanzee	Human
Immune System	mouse	mouse	human	chimpanzee	human
HCV infection	unknown	entry only	+	+	+
HCV pathogenesis	unknown	none	evidence for fibrosis	milder than in humans	fibrosis, cirrhosis, liver cancer
Genetic manipulations	+++	+++	+/-	-	-
Throughput	+++	+++	+/-	+/-	+/-
Costs	+	+	++	++++	+++++
Therapeutics development	unknown	(Vaccines), entry inhibitors	Inhibitors, no vaccines	all classes	all classes

tetraspanin CD81; and two tight junction proteins, claudin-1 and occludin (OCLN). The inability of HCV to efficiently engage at least two of these factors, CD81 and OCLN, precludes entry into murine cells. Using an unbiased selection approach, it was recently demonstrated that a laboratory strain of HCV could be adapted to the mouse CD81 orthologue.[1] The virus acquired mutations in its envelope proteins (E1/E2), which allowed for engagement of the entry factor from mice and other rodents with similar efficiency as human CD81. In addition to modified tropism for CD81, the virus showed altered usage of other HCV entry factors, human SCARB1 and OCLN. Thus, the adaptive mutations appeared to affect the overall HCV envelope confirmation, which raises questions about differences in the entry process of the adapted virus versus naturally occurring HCV. It remains to be shown whether mouse-adapted HCV can infect murine hepatocytes or mice *in vivo*.

Overcoming species barriers with a few adaptive mutations is an exciting precedent. Together with increasing knowledge of the determinants of replication, this study provides the basis for generating an adapted virus that can infect mice. However, testing neutralizing antibodies in this system might be misleading because of conformational differences in the adapted E1/E2 complex. In addition, therapeutics targeting human entry factors would be difficult to test. Nonetheless, an immunocompetent small-

animal model based on a murine-tropic virus strain would be a milestone in HCV research.

Xenotransplantation models for HCV

About a decade ago, it was first demonstrated that mice can be rendered susceptible to HCV infection by engraftment of human hepatocytes. To prevent rejection of the human cells, xenorecipients must be immunocompromised. Recipients are also engineered with an endogenous liver injury, providing a growth stimulus to the usually quiescent hepatocytes and giving the transplanted human cells a competitive advantage. Among the best-characterized liver injury models is the urokinase plasminogen activator (uPA) transgenic (tg) mouse. Liver-specific expression of the uPA transgene is acutely hepatotoxic and severely impairs blood coagulation, which results in high neonatal mortality. Although high levels of human hepatocyte chimerism can be achieved, this model is frail and low in throughput, which has limited its utility.[2] In search of a more robust human liver–chimeric model, mice with a targeted disruption in the fumarylacetoacetate hydrolase gene ($Fah^{-/-}$) were backcrossed to a severely immunocompromised background. *Fah* deficiency is neonatally lethal, but knockout animals can be pharmacologically rescued by administration of the 4-hydroxyphenyl pyruvate dioxygenase inhibitor (2-[2-nitro-4-fluoromethylbenzoyl]-1,3-cyclohexanedione; NTBC); in turn, liver injury can be induced at will by withdrawal of the drug. These animals can be engrafted to high levels with human hepatocytes.[3–5] Both human liver chimeric models have proven useful for the study of human hepatotropic infections *in vivo*. They are also increasingly valued for assessing the preclinical efficacy of drug candidates and for pharmaco-toxicological analyses.

As an alternative to expansion of human hepatocytes in the murine parenchyma, three-dimensional hepatocyte organoids can be transplanted ectopically into immunodeficient xenorecipients.[6] Although such engineered mice have not yet been shown to be susceptible to hepatotropic pathogens, they have the potential to overcome issues of variability in hepatocyte repopulation. High-level liver chimerism has been convincingly demonstrated using primary adult hepatocytes. Stem cell–derived hepatocytes may be an attractive alternative, as they are a renewable resource. Although protocols are being continuously refined to drive human embryonic or induced pluripotent stem cells toward the hepatic lineage, the resulting hepatocyte-like cells do not respond to the same growth stimuli and do not efficiently engraft in current liver injury models. Efforts are ongoing to overcome this barrier, as human liver–chimeric mice engrafted with patient-specific hepatocytes would open unprecedented opportunities to functionally dissect the host genetics of HCV infection.

A major drawback of human liver chimeric mice is their lack of a functional immune system. This is particularly relevant for studies of HCV pathogenesis, as an ongoing inflammatory response is thought to contribute to disease progression. Thus, it would be desirable to dually engraft a donor-matched human liver and (portions of) a human hematopoietic system. Proof-of-concept for this approach was recently provided. AFC8 tg mice express a caspase 8–FK506 binding protein fusion under the control of a liver-specific albumin promoter, and undergo liver injury upon injection of a dimerizer that triggers apoptosis. AFC8 tg mice crossed to a highly immunodeficient background can be reconstituted with human hepatocytes and components of a human immune system. This is achieved by cotransplantation of a mix of donor-matched human hematopoietic progenitor cells, human fetal hepatoblasts, and other nonparenchymal cells. The dually engrafted mice can be infected with HCV and allow the study

of HCV-specific T cells and inflammation.[7] Similar models may be useful to study clinically relevant coinfections with other human-tropic viruses, such as HBV and HIV. The study of human immune responses against HCV replicating in human hepatocytes is a big step forward, yet hurdles remain. Reconstitution is extremely time consuming, requires survival surgery, and is subject to significant donor-to-donor variations. Furthermore, this model does not yet yield predictive results that can be extrapolated to human cohorts.

Genetic host adaptation to study HCV

An inbred, genetically modified mouse model with inheritable susceptibility to HCV would overcome the technical difficulties of xenotransplantation. However, the molecular determinants governing HCV species tropism remain mostly opaque. In murine cells, the viral life cycle is blocked at multiple steps. A clue as to the entry block was provided when CD81 and OCLN were identified as the minimal set of human factors required to render rodent cells permissive to infection *in vitro*.[8] On the basis of this discovery, we constructed a genetically humanized mouse transiently expressing the human entry factors via adenoviral delivery.[9] Using a reporter gene (e.g., luciferase or fluorescent protein) responsive to activation by HCV-encoded CRE recombinase, we showed that viral entry could be detected *in vivo*. This opens up opportunities to genetically dissect HCV uptake in a physiological environment. We established precedent for this by demonstrating the first direct evidence that SCARB1 is a *bona fide* HCV entry factor *in vivo*. Importantly, the genetically humanized mouse is fully immunocompetent, providing the first small animal platform suitable for combined immunization and challenge studies.

Unfortunately, the current model is limited to HCV entry. The ability to reproduce HCV replication and virion assembly/release in mice would dramatically facilitate studies of the life cycle and immune responses. HCV can be coaxed to replicate in murine cells, albeit to very low levels, using recombinant genomes expressing a dominant selectable marker. These studies suggest that all essential host factors for RNA replication are present, but that the murine orthologues may not interact efficiently with the viral proteins. HCV replicates more robustly in mouse cells with a blunted type I interferon response, suggesting that vector-mediated immune activation may limit infection. Stable expression of entry factors in the form of tg or knockin mice would overcome this caveat and may allow identification of a murine background conducive for viral RNA replication. Later stages in the HCV life cycle are likely to be supported in mice, as it was recently reported that infectious particles can assemble in murine hepatoma cell lines.[10]

Summary

There have been significant improvements in HCV animal models over the past few years. Each platform has unique features and can be tailored to address important questions in HCV biology. However, the lack of a small-animal model that allows complete HCV replication and in the context a fully functional immune system remains a major hurdle. It is also unclear whether the natural course of HCV infection, including its associated liver pathology, can be recapitulated in mice. An inbred, fully immunocompetent mouse would be an especially valuable platform to prioritize vaccine candidates and to define effective regimens. In the light of a potential ban on chimpanzee experiments, the need for a model that accurately reflects important hallmarks of HCV infection becomes more pressing than ever.

Acknowledgments

The authors thank Drs. Catherine Murray and Charles M. Rice for comments and edits on the manuscript. Work in the laboratory is supported in part by award number RC1DK087193 from the NIDDK, R01AI072613, and U19 AI057266 from the NIAID, by a Center for Translational Science Award Pilot Grant (UL1 RR024143) from the National Center for Research, the National Institutes of Health through the NIH Roadmap for Medical Research (R01 DK085713–01), the Bill and Melinda Gates Foundation, the Starr Foundation, and the Greenberg Medical Institute. A.P. is a recipient of an Astella Young Investigator Award from the Infectious Society of America. M.D. was supported by postdoctoral fellowship from the German Research Foundation (Deutsche Forschungsgesellschaft).

Conflicts of interest

The authors declare no conflicts of interest.

References

1. Bitzegeio, J. *et al.* 2010. Adaptation of hepatitis C virus to mouse CD81 permits infection of mouse cells in the absence of human entry factors. *PLoS Pathog.* **6:** e1000978.
2. Mercer, D.F. *et al.* 2001. Hepatitis C virus replication in mice with chimeric human livers. *Nat. Med.* **7:** 927–933.
3. Azuma, H. *et al.* 2007. Robust expansion of human hepatocytes in Fah-/-/Rag2-/-/Il2rg-/- mice. *Nat. Biotechnol.* **25:** 903–910.
4. Bissig, K.D. *et al.* 2007. Repopulation of adult and neonatal mice with human hepatocytes: a chimeric animal model. *Proc. Natl. Acad. Sci. U. S. A.* **104:** 20507–20511.
5. Bissig, K.D. *et al.* 2010. Human liver chimeric mice provide a model for hepatitis B and C virus infection and treatment. *J. Clin. Invest.* **120:** 924–930.
6. Chen, A.A. *et al.* 2011. Humanized mice with ectopic artificial liver tissues. *Proc. Natl. Acad. Sci. U. S. A.* **108:** 11842–11847.
7. Washburn, M.L. *et al.* 2011. A humanized mouse model to study hepatitis C virus infection, immune response, and liver disease. *Gastroenterology* **140:** 1334–1344.
8. Ploss, A. *et al.* 2009. Human occludin is a hepatitis C virus entry factor required for infection of mouse cells. *Nature* **457:** 882–886.
9. Dorner, M. *et al.* 2011. A genetically humanized mouse model for hepatitis C virus infection. *Nature* **474:** 208–211.
10. Long, G. *et al.* 2011. Mouse hepatic cells support assembly of infectious hepatitis C virus particles. *Gastroenterology* **141:** 1057–1066.

Ann. N.Y. Acad. Sci. ISSN 0077-8923

ANNALS OF THE NEW YORK ACADEMY OF SCIENCES
Issue: *Animal Models: Their Value in Predicting Drug Efficacy and Toxicity*

Animal models got you puzzled?: think pig

Eric M. Walters,[1,2] Yuksel Agca,[3] Venkataseshu Ganjam,[4] and Tim Evans[3]

[1]National Swine Resource and Research Center, University of Missouri, Columbia, Missouri. [2]Division of Animal Sciences, College of Agriculture Food and Natural Resources, Columbia, Missouri. [3]Department of Veterinary Pathobiology, College of Veterinary Medicine, University of Missouri, Columbia, Missouri. [4]Department of Biomedical Sciences, College of Veterinary Medicine, University of Missouri, Columbia, Missouri

Address for correspondence: Eric M. Walters, Division of Animal Sciences, College of Agriculture Food and Natural Resources, University of Missouri, S134b ASRC 920 E. Campus Dr, Columbia, MO 65211. walterse@missouri.edu

Swine are an excellent large animal model for human health and disease because their size and physiology are similar to humans, in particular, with respect to the skin, heart, gastrointestinal tract, and kidneys. In addition, the pig has many emerging technologies that will only enhance the development of the pig as the nonrodent biomedical model of choice.

Keywords: pig; genetically modified; genome; toxicology; vinclozolin

Animal models are fundamental for insight into the pathogenesis of human diseases and the development of new drugs and predicting their efficacy and toxicity. Classical rodent models have provided valuable information for basic biology; however, one of the disadvantages of the rodent model is the limited ability to sufficiently represent the human disease or syndrome. With similarities between pigs and humans, technology, procedures, and novel treatments developed for human diseases can be applied to swine, and vice versa. Swine have been accepted as the model of choice for applications such as xenotransplantation and surgical training for medical students, as well as for human risk assessment involving the bioavailability environmental contaminants in soil matrices. Spontaneous mutants have also been shown to be valuable experimental models for discovery of molecular mechanisms of human diseases. In the pig, there has been identification of quantitative trait loci for cutaneous melanoma,[1] and a novel mutation (Arg to Cys) in the Low-density lipoprotein (LDL) receptor, which influences spontaneous hypercholesterolemia.[2] Furthermore, pig models have identified additional markers for puerperal psychosis[3] and for human melanocytic proliferation (i.e., RACK1 as a marker of malignancy).[4] Genetically engineered pigs provide a new level of practicality for the biomedical community. With the improvement of the techniques to produce targeted genetic modifications, not only have the number of genetically engineered pigs increased, but also has the number of different diseases models.

Compared to other nonrodent species, the pig is an advantageous animal model to understand human biology, as the structure and function of the pig cardiac vasculature and the gastrointestinal tract, as well as the morphology and physiology of the pig pancreas, are similar to that in humans.[5] However, a relatively minor structural difference between humans and pigs exists within the lymphatic system, where, interestingly, the cortex and medulla of the typical swine lymph node is reversed compared to the human lymph node.[6]

With all of the similarities and a good understanding of the differences between humans and swine, the pig is becoming the nonrodent species of choice for toxicology studies, as they have shown specific responses to a variety of drugs and chemicals that can be administrated by various methods. Moreover, samples can be routinely collected during the dosing period before euthanasia. One other driving force for the use of the pig as a biomedical model for toxicology is the so-called "3Rs"— replacement, reduction, and refinement—as there is a need to resolve inconsistencies between rat and mouse models, and there is increasing societal concern about

doi: 10.1111/j.1749-6632.2011.06345.x

the use of nonhuman primate and canine models. Another property of the pig that is advantageous—but sometimes a disadvantage too—is its size, which is similar to humans. The increase in size relative to rodent models, however, requires the use of more experimental reagents, which can increase costs. This disadvantage is being addressed by the utilization of miniature swine, refinement of porcine-to-murine xenografting procedures, and many other technologies, such as genomics,[7] proteomics, metabalomics, and transgenics in combination with somatic cell nuclear transfer.[8]

The pig will be a novel animal model for studying the potential effects of putative endocrine-disrupting compounds (EDCs) and xenoestrogenic compounds. Little is known about the effects of EDCs on reproductive function in nonrodent species. The hypothesis is that subacute oral exposure to vinclozolin would adversely affect reproductive parameters in the boar. With the potential financial and logistical concerns associated with the use of porcine models in comparative toxicology, we are using testicular tissue xenografting as a novel bioassay, with the aim that porcine-to-murine testicular xenografts can be used as a bioassay. In addition, prepubertal gilts may be used to develop a noninvasive model to evaluate the effects of xenoestrogens. There is evidence that gilts treated with increasing doses of soybean-based phytoestrogens can alter the reproductive tract compared to controls.[9] The results of several studies demonstrate the usefulness and sensitivity of porcine models for studying the adverse effects of endocrine-disrupting chemicals and xenoestrogenic compounds.

The potential use of the pig as the nonrodent biomedical model of choice for toxicology studies could dramatically affect the scientific community. Furthermore, the completion of the swine genome combined with novel techniques, such as cell-based transgenesis, will only enhance the continued use and development of swine as models of human health, syndromes, and conditions. The

National Institutes of Health has established the National Swine Research and Resource Center to better understand human health and to help meet the needs of the biomedical community. The resources at the National Swine Resource and Research Center (www.nsrrc.missouri.edu) are available to aid investigators with their swine needs for biomedical research whether through genetic modification or aid in the development of toxicology studies.

Conflicts of interest

The authors declare no conflicts of interest.

References

1. Du, Z.Q., S. Vincent-Naulleau, H. Gilbert, *et al.* 2007. Detection of novel quantitative trait loci for cutaneous melanoma by genome-wide scan in the MeLiM swine model. *Int. J. Cancer* **120:** 303–320.
2. Grunwald, K.A., K. Schueler, P.J. Uelmen, *et al.* 1999. Identification of a novel Arg–>Cys mutation in the LDL receptor that contributes to spontaneous hypercholesterolemia in pigs. *J. Lipid Res.* **40:** 475–485.
3. Quilter, C.R., C.L. Gilbert, G.L. Oliver, *et al.* 2008. Gene expression profiling in porcine maternal infanticide: a model for puerperal psychosis. *Am. J. Med. Genet. B Neuropsychiatr. Genet.* **147B:** 1126–1137.
4. Egidy, G., S. Jule, P. Bosse, *et al.* 2008. Transcription analysis in the MeLiM swine model identifies RACK1 as a potential marker of malignancy for human melanocytic proliferation. *Mol. Cancer* **7:** 34–45.
5. Larsen, M.O. & B. Rolin. 2004. Use of the Gottingen minipig as a model of diabetes, with special focus on type 1 diabetes research. *ILAR. J.* **45:** 303–313.
6. Johnson, D.K., E.R. Wisner, S.M. Griffey, *et al.* 1996. Sinclair miniature swine melanoma as a model for evaluating novel lymphography contrast agents. In *Advances in Swine in Biomedical Research.* M.E. Tumbleson & L. Schook, Eds.: 607–612. Plenum Press. New York.
7. Archibald, A., L. Bolund, C. Churcher, *et al.* 2010. Pig genome sequence – analysis and publication strategy. *BMC Genomics* **11:** 438–442.
8. Whyte, J.J. & R.S. Prather. 2011. Genetic modifications of pigs for medicine and agriculture. *Mol. Reprod. Dev.* **78:** 879–891.
9. Ford, J.A., S.G. Clark, E.M. Walters, *et al.* 2006. Estrogenic effects of genistein on reproductive tissues of ovariectomized gilts. *J. Anim. Sci.* **84:** 834–842.